Healing Miracles
Great and Small

*Living Proof of
the Success
of Alternative Medicine*

Kennon Rude, D.C.

Trafford Publishing

The ideas, suggestions, and techniques contained in this book are not intended as a substitute for the advice of a health-care practitioner. All matters regarding your physical health should be supervised by a trained professional. Neither the author nor the publisher shall be held responsible for any negative effects resulting from the use of the information described within.

Grateful acknowledgment is made to Louis Sportelli, D.C., for permission to reprint the illustration of the spine from *Introduction to Chiropractic,* by Louis Sportelli, D.C., Copyright 1978.

Names and identifying characteristics of people in the book have been changed to protect the privacy of the individuals.

Editor: Sandra Jonas
Book design: SJ Literary Services
Cover photograph: Joseph P. Jonas III
Cover design: Kuba Holuj

© Copyright 2005 Kennon Rude, D.C.

All rights reserved. No part of this publication may be reproduced, stored in a retrieval system, or transmitted, in any form or by any means, electronic, mechanical, photocopying, recording, or otherwise, without the written prior permission of the author.

Note for Librarians: a cataloguing record for this book that includes Dewey Decimal Classification and US Library of Congress numbers is available from the Library and Archives of Canada. The complete cataloguing record can be obtained from their online database at:
www.collectionscanada.ca/amicus/index-e.html
ISBN 1-4120-3467-1
Printed in Victoria, BC, Canada

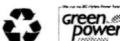

Printed on paper with minimum 30% recycled fibre. Trafford's print shop runs on "green energy" from solar, wind and other environmentally-friendly power sources.

TRAFFORD

Offices in Canada, USA, Ireland and UK

This book was published *on-demand* in cooperation with Trafford Publishing. On-demand publishing is a unique process and service of making a book available for retail sale to the public taking advantage of on-demand manufacturing and Internet marketing. On-demand publishing includes promotions, retail sales, manufacturing, order fulfilment, accounting and collecting royalties on behalf of the author.

Book sales for North America and international:
Trafford Publishing, 6E–2333 Government St.,
Victoria, BC v8t 4p4 CANADA
phone 250 383 6864 (toll-free 1 888 232 4444)
fax 250 383 6804; email to orders@trafford.com
Book sales in Europe:
Trafford Publishing (UK) Ltd., Enterprise House, Wistaston Road Business Centre,
Wistaston Road, Crewe, Cheshire cw2 7rp UNITED KINGDOM
phone 01270 251 396 (local rate 0845 230 9601)
facsimile 01270 254 983; orders.uk@trafford.com
Order online at:
trafford.com/04-1295

10 9 8 7 6 5

*In loving memory of my grandparents,
both of whom were chiropractors,
Elizabeth and William Watts*

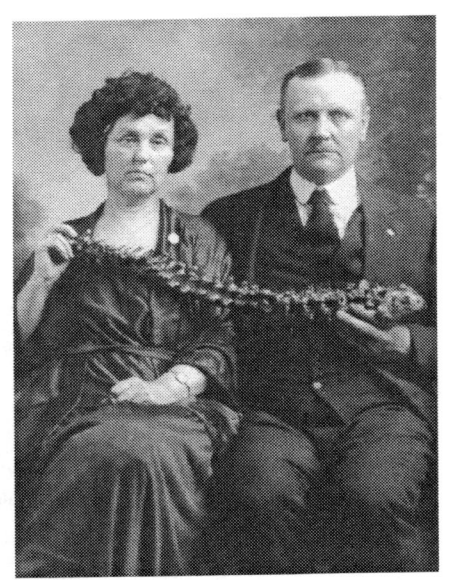

Contents

Foreword ix
Acknowledgments xiii
About This Book xv
Chiropractic Terms xvi
The Spine xvii

1	Introduction: *Tonsillitis and Therapeutic Gems* 1
2	Smitty's Hiccups: *Instant Relief* 5
3	A Little Boy's Crossed Eye: *Normal Vision Restored* 9
4	Mr. Dodd's Third Heart Attack: *Preventive Measures* 13
5	Our Two Babies: *Prenatal Chiropractic Care* 21
6	Herb's Dislocated Shoulder: *Early Intervention* 25
7	The Story of Gigi: *Chiropractic for Animals* 29
8	Barb's Babies: *A Remedy for Miscarriage* 33
9	Dr. Roush's Comments: *Not a Placebo* 38
10	A Flower Child: *From Sinus Infection to Diarrhea* 41
11	An Unusual Shoulder Problem: *Flat Feet* 46
12	The Bed-Wetting Secret: *Embarrassing Problem Solved* ... 54
13	Susan's Ideal Complexion: *Healing Without a Scar* 59
14	Excruciating Eyeball Pain: *Introduction to Cranial Adjustments* 63
15	The Big Fat Guy in the Reception Room: *A Case of High Triglycerides* 70
16	Eva's Congestive Heart Failure: *Miracles Do Happen* 76

CONTENTS

17	Betty's Double Vision: *It Begins with the Neck*	85
18	A Tale of Two Classes: *Chiropractic and Longevity*	90
19	I'm All Pooped Out: *One Solution to Chronic Fatigue*	94
20	Grandpa's Hands: *Learning from the Masters*	101
21	Opal's Toothache: *The Wonders of Acupuncture*	107
22	Ursula and the Pill: *A Little Bit of Humor*	112
23	Pesky Nail Fungus: *A Different Approach*	115
24	Chronic Motion Sickness: *A Simple Remedy*	123
25	Harry's Hay Fever: *Secondary Benefits*	127
26	Evelyn's Calcific Bursitis: *Chemistry Comes to the Rescue*	134
27	Ruby's Poor Old Back: *Surgery Is Not the Only Answer*	138
28	Amanda's Herpes: *Treating Skepticism, Headaches, and Cold Sores*	144
29	Samantha's Sciatica: *Delving Deeper to Find the Cause*	153
30	Water in the Ear, a Broken Rib, and Sunburn: *Seeing Is Believing*	158
Epilogue		165
Appendix		167
Complimentary Chiropractic Visit		169

Foreword

Darcy McKinstry-Truppo, the former executive secretary of the Colorado Chiropractic Association, asked me to introduce my friend Dr. Kennon Rude to his readers. I am flattered that she considered me competent enough to record the many fine qualities of one of the best chiropractors I have ever known.

I met Dr. Rude in 1981 shortly after graduating from Logan College of Chiropractic in Missouri and moving to Denver. I had set up a meeting with Dr. Donald Zisch, a longtime Denver chiropractor and the president of the Logan Alumni Association, to gather information about state chiropractic laws and the best places to practice. Dr. Zisch insisted Dr. Rude be included because "he is *the* one who can fill you in on all the important things you should know." When Dr. Rude accepted our invitation, I was very impressed that a doctor would agree to spend time advising a fresh-out-of-college neophyte. Upon meeting him, I knew I was in the presence of a warmhearted and devoted healer, one with a vast knowledge of chiropractic and alternative medicine. He quickly became my friend and mentor.

Kennon Rude hails from a long line of chiropractors. He was born to chiropractic parents *and* chiropractic maternal grandparents on July 5, 1923, in Bemidji, Minnesota. Initially, he chose to study chemical engineering when he entered the University of Minnesota in the fall of 1941. After World War II began in December of that year, Kennon was called to serve by the U.S. Navy to meet a demand for engineers. The navy's college training program allowed him to continue his engineering studies before going into active duty. On his birthday in 1945, he was commissioned ensign, and after serving as an engineering officer aboard two ships, he was honorably discharged in 1946.

It was his grandfather's passion for chiropractic—and his impending retirement—that propelled Kennon to change his career

FOREWORD

direction and follow in his family's footsteps. In January 1947 he enrolled at National Chiropractic College in Chicago, the only college at that time offering full-body dissection in the anatomy department. He later transferred to Northwestern College of Chiropractic in Minneapolis, from which he graduated in 1950. Within a few days of graduation, he received his license to practice and joined his parents at the Rude Chiropractic Center in Hector, Minnesota.

Kennon likes to tell a story about how he promoted his business in its early years: An attorney friend was starting a practice in Hector and decided to file for the office of county attorney. Kennon asked him, "Bill, why are you filing for county attorney? You've been in the county for less than six months. Nobody even knows there *is* a Bill Sutor, attorney-at-law." Bill replied, "That's the point exactly. I pay a filing fee of only twenty-four dollars, and all the voters will at least find out I exist." Thinking that was a great way to inexpensively publicize his name, Kennon filed for county coroner. And sure enough, he was elected. He served as Renville County Coroner for four years (1954–1958). Also during his years in Minnesota, he was the chairman for the American Red Cross, teaching first aid to many of the people in the county. And as an instructor for the course based on Dale Carnegie's book *How to Win Friends and Influence People,* he taught human relations subjects throughout southern Minnesota.

After providing the Hector community with chiropractic and alternative health care for almost twenty years, Kennon moved his family and practice to Boulder, Colorado, in late 1969. Just a few months later, he opened the Boulder Chiropractic Center and has continued serving the Boulder area to this day.

Throughout his many years in practice, he has been a continuous learner, taking numerous courses. His late wife, Shirley, used to refer to him as a professional student. His postgraduate studies have included chiropractic orthopedics, chiropractic radiology, acupuncture, methods of pain control modification, and sports injuries. In 1974 he earned a B.S. degree in bionutrition from Columbia College in Missouri. Under the statutes of both Minnesota and Colorado, Doctors of Chiropractic must complete at least 15 hours of postgraduate study annually to renew their licenses. Considering Dr. Rude's fifty-five-year career, that requirement has led to an equivalent of 825 hours of postgraduate work, or about fifty-five semesters.

His other great accomplishments include a U.S. patent for a cervical traction device, participation in the founding of the American Chiropractic Association Council of Sports Injuries, and the Chiropractor of the Year Award in 1980.

Kennon cares deeply for his patients. He will never refuse anyone treatment, regardless of an inability to pay. And his mind is always active, correlating physical symptoms with something he may have learned years ago. Consequently, he is continuously developing innovative procedures to solve health problems. He strives to discover more about natural ways to correct the "dis-eases" that grip his patients. I, along with many of the chiropractors in Boulder, consult with him when we have difficult cases, or for our own personal care.

Dr. Rude has taught me a great deal. I consider myself blessed to have known and worked with him throughout the years. You can benefit also by reading his tales of alternative healing success stories.

Bill White
Doctor of Chiropractic

Acknowledgments

I would like to express my utmost gratitude to the patients whose health problems are presented in this book. Rather than turning to orthodox medicine, they trusted my expertise in alternative health care. In some cases, the traditional approach had failed, and my treatment was a last resort. Suffice it to say that my writing of this volume is a great big THANK YOU! to all of my patients over the last fifty-five years.

I would like to acknowledge that I am not the great healer who performs miracles. I believe a power far greater than any living being is responsible for restoring the ailing body. I simply act as a conduit for the collection and dissemination of information about a patient's problem so the unhealthy condition can be restored to normal. I have often made the statement, "Someone up there looks after me." To this power I am truly grateful.

I want to extend a special thank-you to the individuals who have helped me record these tales of alternative healing:

My late wife, Shirley, who was able to see only the beginnings of this composition before her sudden death in 1998. The fact that I could lose myself in writing was a godsend in my grieving process.

Sandra Jonas, whose writing and editing genius—and talents for book layout and design—proved invaluable. Her persistence and patience are second to none, and I thank her for keeping me on course throughout the revision process.

Four chiropractors—Drs. Richard Tyler, Herrick de Charette, Karl Nealer, and Bill White—who all played a major role in the evolution of this work.

Jeanmarie MacKelvey, whom I met through the Social Singles Club of Boulder, for her unwavering encouragement and support in helping me complete this tome.

My patient Dave Wilson, who urged me to invest in a computer.

ACKNOWLEDGMENTS

All of the patients at the Associated Boulder Chiropractors Wellness Center who read each chapter as I finished it and helped with the initial proofreading.

And the many individuals who taught me the science, art, and philosophy of chiropractic—not only the professors at National Chiropractic College and Northwestern College of Chiropractic, but also my parents and mother's parents. To them I am especially indebted. Without their support, I probably would have become a chemical engineer, and I never would have experienced the wonderful joys and rewards from healing others.

About This Book

To convey my message about alternative health care most effectively, I chose a form of communication as old as language itself: storytelling. Far more engaging and entertaining than academic writing, stories are ideal for presenting new or complicated concepts.

I've made every effort to simplify the information presented without sacrificing what I hoped to relay. Unavoidably, however, I had to intersperse the narratives with medical terms. The first time they're mentioned in each chapter, they are italicized and followed by definitions or explanations. In addition, since I rely heavily on chiropractic in my practice, I've frequently used chiropractic terms, the most common of which are listed and defined at the front of the book. Appreciating that a picture is worth a thousand words, I have also included a detailed diagram of the spine. I recommend reviewing this information before diving into the stories, returning back to it as needed.

Although most of the chapters are self-contained, I urge you to read *Healing Miracles Great and Small* cover to cover the first time through to gain a firm understanding of chiropractic and other non-traditional therapies. After that, the page headings corresponding to the health problem discussed in the text below will make it easy to flip back to a section that addresses your particular situation. Also, I introduce a number of nutritional supplements and alternative therapies—see the appendix for a list of sources and contacts.

At the back of *Healing Miracles Great and Small* are instructions for obtaining a complimentary visit to a chiropractor. Please take advantage of this opportunity. My goal is to help you achieve the significant health benefits I have been able to offer my patients.

Chiropractic Terms

adjusting table. A specially designed low-to-the-floor cushioned table with an opening for the face to allow the patient's spine to lie in a straight line, parallel to the floor.

cervical. Relating to the seven vertebrae in the neck, designated by C1–C7.

chiropractic. Established as a profession in 1895, this science is based on the premise that good health depends on a normal functioning nervous system. Misalignments of the spinal bones can interfere with nerve impulses and cause a wide variety of ailments. Without relying on drugs, chiropractors restore good health by using adjustment and manipulation techniques to align the spine.

dis-ease. Term originated more than a century ago by David D. Palmer, the founder of chiropractic, to describe malfunctions of the body.

lumbar. Relating to the five vertebrae in the lower back, designated by L1–L5.

palpate. Using the fingers to examine for misalignments by gently pressing between two vertebrae and comparing their positions.

sacral. Relating to the five fused vertebrae located in the pelvis area, designated by S1–S5.

spinal adjustment. The application of short and sharp, but gentle, thrusts to misaligned vertebrae to move them back to their proper positions.

subluxation. A misaligned, or displaced, joint.

thoracic. Relating to the twelve vertebrae in the midback region, designated by T1–T12.

vertebra, *pl.* **vertebrae.** One of the thirty-three bones forming the spinal column, divided into seven cervical, twelve thoracic, five lumbar, five sacral, and four coccygeal.

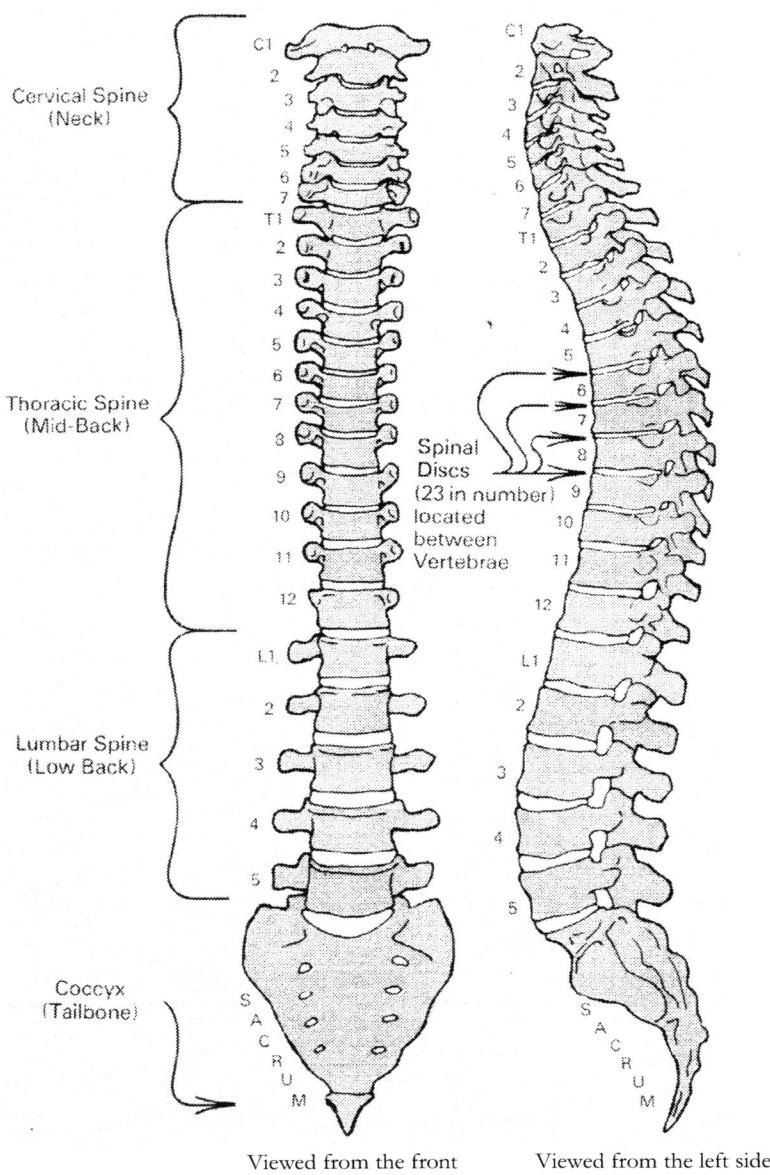

The Spine

1

Introduction
Tonsillitis and Therapeutic Gems

> The doctor of the future will give no medicine but will interest his patients in the care of the human frame, in diet, and in the cause and prevention of disease.
>
> *Thomas Edison*

As a Doctor of Chiropractic for fifty-five years, I have had the good fortune to help heal hundreds of patients. Some of them I saw only briefly, while others I have known for decades, treating them and later treating their children. Their success stories stand as proof of the effectiveness of alternative, holistic care. Beginning nearly twenty years ago, a series of events convinced me it was time to record their stories. And in sharing their healing triumphs, I hope that others may benefit as well.

The impetus for this collection resides in a 1987 issue of *Dynamic Chiropractic*, a bimonthly publication that reports the latest news in the field of chiropractic. This journal also features several columns about pertinent subjects that interest chiropractors, such as nutrition, acupuncture, x-ray, rehabilitation, and practice management.

In the August 15 issue, a column by Dr. Richard Tyler, titled "A Therapeutic Gem," describes a nonmedical, all-natural regimen for acute tonsillitis. He outlines the relationship between the nerves of the upper *cervical* area (top of the neck) and the tissues of the throat, and explains how chiropractic adjustments in this area can stimulate the body's life force to promote healing. Dr. Tyler also details a simple method by which a doctor, using a gloved finger, can extricate the cheesy, pus-like substance from the crypts of the infected tonsillar tissues. The accumulation of this debris and its difficult removal make the management of tonsillitis especially challenging.

I agreed completely with Dr. Tyler's explanation and approach. My grandfather, the first of three generations of chiropractors in my family, had taught me the very same protocol, which I had been using successfully for thirty-five years. Generally, the public doesn't visit a chiropractor for tonsillitis, so Dr. Tyler had done a great service to the profession by explaining that chiropractic is beneficial for much more than common back pains.

Believing a thank-you was in order, I wrote a letter to the editor, commending Dr. Tyler for his excellent article. I included a short paragraph describing the herbal *Wonder Oil* (WO), an effective extract of sage I had added to my treatment of sore throats. With this antiseptic oil on my gloved finger, I massage the tonsil tissue directly, and the throat tenderness diminishes in just five minutes. I then follow with Dr. Tyler's protocol.

I ended my letter by asking the editor to consider incorporating a regular column titled "Therapeutic Gems" to which other doctors could contribute their own tricks of the trade. This information would help practitioners who had not been taught these methods in college. "I could probably write four or five articles about special techniques that have worked for my patients," I added.

Dynamic Chiropractic did publish my letter, and about six months later, I received a long distance call from Dr. Herrick de Charette of Cairns, Australia. He told me he had tried WO as I had described and was thrilled with the excellent results. Eager for more ideas, he asked if I'd be willing to teach him the additional four or five tricks I had mentioned. He was planning to visit America for a Parker Seminar[*] in the upcoming year and requested to meet me at my office in Boulder, Colorado. Flattered, I agreed to see him.

Several months after our conversation, I received a letter from Dr. de Charette detailing his itinerary: He'd be arriving in the United States within three weeks and had scheduled two days in Boulder to

---

[*]First held in 1951, the highly respected Parker Seminars were conceived by James W. Parker, D.C., as a means to provide chiropractors with efficient, successful methods for improving and promoting their practices.

learn about my therapeutic gems. Uh-oh, now I was on the spot. Since I had boasted about having a number of ideas, I *had* to deliver. So I started a list. Every time I treated a patient with an unusual method, I wrote it down. Soon I had thirteen pearls of wisdom, and the number continued to grow. By the time Dr. de Charette arrived, I had recorded twenty-two. After sharing all of them with my grateful colleague, I decided to maintain the list and have consistently added to it.

Almost a decade later, I joined Drs. Karl Nealer and Bill White in a conversation about the demands insurance companies and managed care organizations had placed on chiropractic. I remember Bill said, "Kenn, you were in practice long before chiropractic was ever included in insurance coverage. Back in those days, patients paid cash for your services, happy to pay for remedies that medical doctors couldn't offer."

"You're right," I said. "I took care of just about any kind of problem that walked through the front door. Today, chiropractic colleges emphasize musculoskeletal conditions and are not teaching some of the techniques I learned in school. The general public believes a chiropractor addresses only back problems, whiplash, or maybe a headache. Typically, very few people go to a chiropractor for acute tonsillitis or other non-back-related problems."

To illustrate my point, I produced my list of therapeutic gems, at that time numbering in the high eighties. After scanning the list, Karl looked up and said, "I have a great idea! Write a book and explain your treatment for each condition. As more and more research is being done, the chiropractic knowledge database is expanding so fast that educators have to ignore subjects that were taught years ago. Young doctors just don't learn this information—it would be a shame if all of it were lost."

"Hey, you're on to something," Bill said, taking the list from Karl, "but I think you need to broaden the scope of the book to include the average lay person—not just chiropractors or students. There are millions of people suffering from all types of health problems, and you could give them the chance to learn about alternative approaches."

Inspired by their enthusiasm, I began to document the many ailments I've resolved with nontraditional techniques. *Healing Miracles*

Great and Small is a compilation of those cases, written in an easy-to-read story format. In general, each chapter presents a true narrative of one patient, the illness or complaint, and the corresponding treatment.

I chose not to present the stories in a chronological fashion, instead ordering them according to the ailment and the type of treatment introduced. I occasionally bounce back and forth between Hector, Minnesota, where I began my practice, and Boulder, Colorado, where I practice today.

My objective in writing *Healing Miracles* is threefold: (1) to encourage lay readers to take responsibility for their health and seek out chiropractic and other highly effective nontraditional therapies; (2) to show both patients and doctors the wide variety of conditions that respond to alternative, conservative, and noninvasive holistic care; and (3) to record for posterity numerous time-tested methods that can augment any physician's patient-management skills.

In looking back over the many years, amidst the joys and frustrations of the healing process, I realized I never stopped learning from my patients. I urge you to do the same—listen with an open mind to their stories so you, too, can learn about healing yourself, your patients, or loved ones.

2

Smitty's Hiccups
Instant Relief

> Depending upon your age and how many years you practice, you will perform a number of miracles with your hands.
> *J.J. Janse, D.C.*
> *President, National College of Chiropractic*

During one of my first classes at National College of Chiropractic in the late 1940s, Dr. J.J. Janse discussed the basic tenets of the chiropractic philosophy of healing. I was already acquainted with these truths, having grown up in a family in which both parents as well as maternal grandparents were chiropractors. Dr. Janse's message was a familiar one; namely, chiropractors strive to locate the cause of an ailment, and after removing that cause, they trust in the body's natural ability to heal itself. He concluded by summarizing the five fundamentals underlying this remarkable science:

1. A vertebra can become *subluxated* (misaligned).

2. Radiating out from the spinal cord through the opening between the subluxated vertebra and the adjacent vertebra is a spinal nerve whose impulses are altered by the subluxation.

3. These atypical nerve impulses may disturb the function of the tissue (skin, muscles, or internal organs) supplied by that spinal nerve (the skin may exhibit numbness or burn-

ing; the muscles, a weakness or spasm; internal organs, reduced or overactive function).

4. Removing the subluxation will restore the nerve to normal function.

5. The tissue that was deprived of normal nerve energy will also return to normal function.

Since my childhood, I've seen these principles at work countless times. Often, a simple adjustment of the vertebra will instantly relieve symptoms. An especially striking example of this happened just a few weeks after Dr. Janse's lecture.

National College had a basketball team, and I'd eagerly signed up to play. At the first practice session I met the starting team: Andy, Bob, Bill, Ray, and Smitty. I joined four others—Kemp, Don, Vern, and our towering six-foot-five center, Keineth—to make up the second string.

At an away game early in the season, the gym had an unusual configuration. One of the baskets was mounted so close to the end wall that there were only about eight inches between the end of the court and a concrete block wall. A heavy wrestling mat hung under the basket to cushion those who ran out of bounds.

Halfway through the game, an opponent fouled Smitty, the point guard who brought the ball down court and set up the plays. Although a bit pudgy, he was nimble footed, making him a great asset to the team.

Smitty stepped up to shoot his free throw. He bounced the ball a few times, paused, took aim, and shot. Despite its graceful arch, the ball struck the front edge of the rim and rebounded back to Smitty who grabbed it and started dribbling toward the basket. As he was charging forward for a layup, an opponent deliberately tripped him, launching his hefty bulk into the air. Smitty crashed headfirst into the wall, bounced off the mat, and then flopped to the floor.

He was out cold.

A few of us dragged an unconscious Smitty to a bench. We laid him down so his head was lower than his body, and in seconds he regained consciousness. Then something very strange happened. As he moved to sit up, he started to hiccup. "Hic . . . hic . . . hic."

A substitute was sent in and the game resumed. Smitty sat to my right, dazed and unsteady, his hiccups continuing nonstop. Obviously he was in distress, but being just a freshman, I had no idea how to help him. I felt powerless.

Our student coach, Ken Ketchum, a senior with much more experience, knew exactly what to do. He stood facing Smitty, bent forward, and starting at the base of the skull and moving downward, used his fingers to *palpate* (touch and press) Smitty's neck bones. Ken felt each vertebra and compared it to the one above and below, checking for any improper alignment. His fingers stopped near the fifth *cervical* vertebra (the midneck region). With Smitty's next hiccup, Ken carefully placed his hands, making a specific contact on the fifth vertebra. He held tight. "Hic." He rotated Smitty's head toward the right. "Hic." Raising Smitty's chin, Ken waited for another hiccup and then gave a short, sharp thrust, adjusting the vertebra. I heard a popping sound, and—

the hiccups stopped.

The following day, I reflected back on Smitty's injury, thinking about how it related to Dr. Janse's lecture:

1. *Subluxated vertebra.* When Smitty ran into the wall, the fifth cervical vertebra was forced out of place.

2. *Alteration of nerve impulses.* There was a change in the impulses of the *phrenic* nerve, a branch of the fifth cervical nerve that emits through the opening between the fifth and sixth cervical vertebra.

3. *Tissue function is altered.* The subluxation in Smitty's neck caused the corresponding tissue at the other end of the phrenic nerve—the diaphragm—to function abnormally, leading to the hiccups.

4. *Removal of subluxation restores nerve function.* When Ken adjusted Smitty's neck, he removed the subluxation at the fifth cervical vertebra (the cause of the problem).

5. *Tissue is returned to normal function.* When the subluxation was corrected, the normal function of the diaphragm was restored, and the hiccups stopped.

So, at the gym the night before, I had actually observed firsthand a demonstration of chiropractor philosophy.

Many times over the last fifty-five years, I've read or heard about some poor individual who has been suffering with hiccups for an extended time, sometimes for weeks or even months. The media often play up the many suggested remedies that have been tried without success. Please remember this: Chiropractic and a simple neck adjustment can bring immediate relief.

3

A Little Boy's Crossed Eye
Normal Vision Restored

> The . . . third cranial nerve is the nerve supply of all the muscles of the eye except the superior oblique and the external rectus. Its primary concern is wholly in supplying motor function or movement to the eyeball. Injury to this nerve may droop the lids, give . . . crossed eyes, or give inability to rotate the eye on its axis. Very often these troubles may be corrected by a good spinal adjustment to the cervical [neck] region, as the nerves from the middle and upper cervical region connect with the [third cranial nerve].
>
> *Joe Shelby Riley, M.D., D.C., D.O., Ph.D.*
> The Science and Practice of Chiropractic, *1925*

On the first day of my practice, September 18, 1950, I joined my parents, Drs. Harold and Beatrice Rude, at the Rude Chiropractic Center in Hector, Minnesota. I spent the morning meeting their patients and observing my father perform adjustments. Toward midday a woman from Hutchinson brought in her five-year-old son for an appointment. She had driven nearly thirty miles (a long trip in those days) to see if my father could help her small boy. Wally was a cute child with dark, wavy hair. The only detraction from his handsome face—and the reason for their visit—was his severely crossed left eye.

Just a few months before, young Wally de Gette had viewed the world through normal eyes. His life changed abruptly one afternoon while he was riding in the car with his dad. Wally sat in the passenger seat as they sped down the highway to pick up his mom at his grandmother's house. They reached the busy interstate where his dad was supposed to stop—but he didn't. Traveling at about fifty-five miles per hour, the car roared through the intersection and smashed into a fully loaded semitrailer. Mr. de Gette died instantly on impact, whereas his son flew through the windshield and miraculously survived.

After spending more than a week in the hospital, Wally returned home to recuperate. Nearly three weeks later, when he seemed almost fully recovered, his left eye began to cross. Alarmed by this strange occurrence, Mrs. de Gette consulted with several medical professionals to determine the cause. An optometrist suggested Wally wear a pair of corrective lenses, while an ophthalmologist (an eye specialist) recommended a surgical procedure for shortening the eye muscles, forcing the eye to straighten. She declined both treatments as neither explained why her son's eye crossed following the accident.

One doctor thought Wally might be emotionally disturbed. Mrs. de Gette took him to a children's psychologist who believed the sight of his dad's death was so distressing that Wally's eye crossed to blur the painful memory. He prescribed an extended period of treatment for a year or two. Mrs. de Gette wasn't convinced. Yes, her husband's death had been a gruesome scene, but Wally hadn't actually *seen* it. On the contrary, he had gone through the windshield and landed unconscious beside the car.

Finally, a friend urged her to take Wally to see Dr. Harold Rude, a chiropractor in Hector, who reportedly had had success with difficult cases. Although three chiropractors practiced in Hutchinson and one in nearby Glencoe, she heeded her friend's advice and drove the extra distance.

My father carefully examined Wally, took x-rays, and then invited me and Mrs. DeGette into his office. "This is what I've found," he said. "The trauma from the accident displaced young Wally's top two cervical vertebrae, C1 and C2, located just below the base of the skull. This abnormal positioning puts considerable twisting stress on the brain stem, which connects to the spinal cord and lies inside the skull. Now, branching off the brain stem are the nerves to the eye muscles—the third, fourth, and sixth cranial nerves. By adjusting the misaligned vertebrae in Wally's neck, I should be able to restore the integrity of both the brain stem and the cranial nerves, allowing them to function properly again. I'm very optimistic that a series of adjustments will correct his crossed eye."

At last, Mrs. de Gette's had received the information she needed to help her son.

I watched my father carefully palpate the boy's two upper cervical vertebrae. Then he precisely placed his hands on Wally's small neck and gave a mild thrust to move the bones in the desired direction.

My father adjusted Wally two to three times a week for a month, coaxing his vertebrae and the surrounding musculature back to their normal positions. By the fifth week, his eye started to return to center. Mrs. de Gette nodded her approval as my dad expressed how well his young patient was responding to treatment.

Wally's eye recovered completely over the next four months of weekly adjustments. I had started seeing my own patients during that time, but I always took a minute to chat with Mrs. de Gette and her son whenever they were in the office. Ultimately, Wally no longer needed treatment, and he and his mom stopped coming to the Rude Center.

Several years later, I received an unexpected phone call. "Dr. Rude, this is Wally de Gette. Do you remember me?"

"Wally de Gette... Of course! How *are* you?"

He filled me in on what he'd been doing since I had last seen him. He'd been quite an athlete in high school, lettering in football, wrestling, and track, so at college he majored in physical education to pursue a career as a sports coach. The curriculum required that he take a course in first aid to prepare him for any injuries during practice or games. Wally passed both levels of training provided by the American Red Cross, qualifying him to be a first aid instructor. After fulfilling all the other requirements, he graduated and accepted a football coaching position in Bird Island, only nine miles west of Hector.

"You know, Wally, early on in my practice, I completed the Red Cross classes too." I had decided that a chiropractor teaching CPR and other aspects of first aid would be an excellent form of public service. As I was the only person in Renville County with the proper training, I was appointed the county's first aid chairman, in charge of the instruction materials. I stored everything in my office basement.

"That's why I called. The Bird Island Fire Department asked me to teach first aid to all the volunteer firemen, and they said I needed to contact you for the visual aids."

I told him to stop by and pick them up, and later that day, he visited the office for the first time in sixteen years. I recognized him immediately: the same wavy hair, the same fetching smile. I stepped forward to greet him.

"Long time, no see," he said.

We sat and reminisced about the car accident and his crossed eye. I told him my folks had both retired about a year earlier. He was disappointed my father wasn't there.

"Has your eye ever bothered you?" I asked.

"No, it's been perfect ever since the last adjustment from your dad. If I'm overtired, I sometimes feel tension around the inside of my eyeball. All I need is some rest, though, and then my eye's okay."

I felt blessed that our paths had crossed again. As I've often said, "Someone up there looks after me." Very few doctors are afforded the opportunity to participate in such an unusual case, let alone be able to follow up so many years later. I believe there was a guiding hand leading Wally's mom to the Rude Center. Her devotion to finding the reason for her son's condition and my father's skills restored Wally's eyesight, allowing him to later become a star athlete and successful coach.

Occasionally, I notice toddlers wearing glasses. Wally comes to mind, and I wonder if the birthing process caused a misalignment in the neck. During delivery, especially a lengthy or difficult one, a tremendous force is placed on the infant's vulnerable neck. I contend that a chiropractic examination for all newborns should be a routine part of postdelivery care. One easy adjustment could remedy a lifetime of vision problems.

4

Mr. Dodd's Third Heart Attack
Preventive Measures

> The heart is so important. It starts to beat before we are born and continues to do so until the moment of our death. Chiropractic can do so much to help heart conditions that I want every Doctor of Chiropractic to know how to take care of heart patients.
>
> *Robert E. Coyler, D.C.*
> *Early Chiropractor Researcher*

After the harsh, drab Minnesota winters, spring's sunshine and colors always put a lilt in my step. It was Mother Nature at one of her finest moments: blades of grass greening the horizon, tiny buds hinting at the trees, and young tulips and crocuses poking through the ground. I remember a beautiful spring morning in 1955 when I literally skipped up the sidewalk and into my office.

"Oh, it's such a beautiful day and good morning to you," I almost burst into song as I greeted Ada, my receptionist.

"G-g-good morning to you too," she stammered, not accustomed to my exuberance.

I went back to the consultation room to read the mail and wait for my first appointment of the day. Just a few minutes later, Ada knocked on the door. "Kenneth Shultz is here to see you," she said.

I was always pleased when Ken stopped by. He represented Standard Process Laboratories, a nutritional supplement manufacturer located in Palmyra, Wisconsin. After finding out about his company and their excellent all-natural products, I became hooked. For more than fifty years, I've used their supplements to help treat all types of illnesses.

Standard Process has always done an excellent job of training and educating their salespeople, and through Ken, I learned a great deal about nutrition. Because Northwestern College of Chiropractic had been in its infancy when I attended, I had received only a basic tutelage in biochemistry.

As with most of his visits, it wasn't long before Ken's favorite subject came up. "So, Kennon," he said, grinning, "is this the day you'll buy an endocardiograph?"

As part of their ongoing research on vitamins and minerals, and how they affect the prevention and cure of various illnesses, Standard Process had introduced the endocardiograph in the late 1930s. Dr. Royal Lee, the company founder, had designed the device, a recording stethoscope that can trace the sounds emitting from the chest wall as the heart muscles contract. He and his colleagues had discovered that changes in body chemistry almost instantly show up in the heart, and therefore the administration of specific nutrients can alter its action. They found, for example, that vitamin B-2 slows *tachycardia* (rapid heart rate), and vitamin B-1 and potassium stabilize *arrythmia* (irregular heart rate). Essentially, the endocardiograph can measure nutritional status, actually using the heart to provide a permanent, detailed recording of a patient's level of health.

"Not a chance," I answered. Ken Shultz had demonstrated the machine to me on several occasions, trying to convince me to use it in my practice. But I'd always turned a negative ear to his sales pitch. I doubted enough people would consider trusting a chiropractor with a heart-measuring device that even medical doctors didn't use. "As I've told you before, Ken, the *electro*cardiograph is the instrument of choice these days, and—"

Ada burst into the room. "Sorry to interrupt, but you'd better come right away. There's a new patient outside. His wife came in first to see if this was the right office. She told me her husband is very weak and might need help getting into the building."

I rushed to the front door just in time to see a woman struggling through with a man leaning heavily on her arm. He dropped into the first chair inside the room and gripped his chest. His sickly pallor worried me. In all my years in practice, I've never seen a patient in worse shape.

"My name's Alma Dodd and this is my husband, Leonard. He thinks he's close to having another heart attack—and he's already had two." She sat down next to him and took a deep breath. "He had the first one three years ago and stayed in the hospital for two and a half weeks. It happened in September, right in the middle of the harvest. Thank goodness our neighbors pitched in to help finish. Come spring, Leonard still wasn't well enough, so we had to rent out the entire farm to two neighbors. But by the *next* spring, the doctor said he was okay and Leonard planted all the crops."

"I guess I tried to do too much," Mr. Dodd managed to say, "because I could feel that same tightness in my chest—just like I felt before my heart attack." He was fighting to breathe. "I went back to Dr. Heinz . . . and he put me in the hospital under observation. . . . It was while I was there that I had my second attack." He turned to his wife.

"Leonard had to give up farming after that," she continued for him. "We hired a neighbor to do all the field work that summer, and then we put the farm into the soil bank." (Because the United States was overproducing grains at that time, the government created the Soil Bank Program to pay farmers for not growing crops.)

"I've got that same heavy feeling in my chest now," Mr. Dodd tried again, "and I get so winded, even with doing practically nothing. I know I'll have another attack if I don't do something different. The doctors didn't prevent the second attack. . . . The owner of the coffee shop in Franklin told us to go to Hector and see Dr. Rude."

An excellent cook, "Ma" Abraham operated a small restaurant just off the main highway that passed to the north of Franklin, Minnesota. Having recovered from chronic constipation under the care of my dad, she referred over a dozen patients from the Franklin area to the Rude Center in Hector.

We all looked over to Ken Schultz as he was making his way through the reception room toward the front door. "Hold on a second, Ken," I said. "Can I speak to you for a minute?"

Back in my office, I got right to the point. "If you ever expect me to buy one of those endocardiographs, you'd better bring one in and do an exam on this patient. He's had two heart attacks in the last three years, and he feels another one coming on."

Without a word, Ken turned, raced outside, and brought in his demo model. After setting it up in an adjusting room, we helped Mr. Dodd into the room and Ken removed his shirt. He applied the microphone to Leonard's chest wall and explained the procedure. When Ken finished, he motioned me into my office. "I think we did this test just in the nick of time," he whispered. "He's in a pre–heart attack state now, and I believe he's only a few hours to a day away from a full-fledged attack. He needs some *Cataplex B*, *Cataplex G*, and *Cardiotrophin* immediately. I'd also add some *Phosfood*."

I hurried to my supplement cabinet and found everything he had recommended—except Cataplex B. I asked Ken if he had any in his car. "Sure thing," he said. "I'll bring in a couple of bottles." I let out a sigh of relief.

Supplements in hand, we returned to the adjusting room. "You were very smart to come in when you did," Ken said, sitting down next to Leonard. "You *are* close to having another attack." Leonard's eyes widened in panic. "Oh, don't worry—you're going to be okay. I suggest these four things right away: This liquid—it's called Phosfood—is mostly phosphorus and tends to thin the blood like aspirin. It'll help prevent your heart attack because thinner blood will pass through the tiny capillaries more easily, reducing any chance of clotting in the coronary arteries. You'll notice a kind of lemon juice taste. Cataplex B, which contains vitamin B-1, helps the nerve conductivity to the heart, and the vitamins B-2 and B-3 in Cataplex G will support the liver, where all the blood must pass through before going to the heart. And Cardiotrophin acts as a heart muscle tonic. It'll help strengthen the heart almost instantly." He removed two tablets from each bottle and handed them to Leonard along with a glass of water containing several drops of Phosfood. "Swallow these pills and then drink all the water," he instructed.

"I'm using vitamins almost like drugs," Ken said, addressing both of us. "That's what nature intended in the first place. Long before pharmacies existed, healers turned to plants for remedies. We know that when the early settlers came to America, the doctors relied on local foods and herbs for treating sickness. Physicians up north used different items from those down south for treating the same ailment.

"When the thirteen colonies started to negotiate the formation of the United States, they sent delegates to the Continental Congress. Most of them were doctors because they were considered the best educated. Naturally, they talked shop as well as politics, and soon they were sending herbs and roots from one area to another. This spawned a new occupation—the druggist—who had supplies from different parts of the country.

"As America grew, scientists began studying the herbs, trying to isolate the ingredients responsible for healing. Pharmaceutical companies appeared on the scene, and eventually they produced those ingredients synthetically to save money. Standard Process Laboratories, however, never joined that bandwagon—we pride ourselves on our pure supplements. The plant sources we use are raised without commercial fertilizers or any other additives that might contaminate them. And the company dates back to 1929, making it one of the oldest manufacturers of nutritional supplements.

"Gee, I better stop talking so Dr. Rude can do a thorough physical exam. I'll talk with you again before you leave."

Leonard thanked Ken and said, "You know, I feel better already. I can breathe a little easier, and that heaviness isn't as bad."

I examined Mr. Dodd as much as he could physically tolerate. The chiropractic spinal exam, the most important part, revealed he had several areas in his spine where normal motion was absent.

"It appears you have other factors contributing to your problem," I told him. "I'd like to take x-rays of your spine and check to see if you have any conditions, like arthritis, that would prevent me from giving you chiropractic adjustments."

As we were completing the x-rays, I saw Leonard was just too exhausted to continue. "I think that's enough for one day," I said. "You go home and rest. Make an appointment for tomorrow, and in the meantime, I'll study your x-rays. Ken will lay out a schedule for taking those supplements. And don't worry about the charge—we'll talk about that next time." I didn't want to add more stress by discussing finances, possibly undoing any positive effects.

I watched as they headed for their car. Mrs. Dodd was not supporting her husband; in fact, he seemed steadier on his feet. Satisfied—and relieved—he was okay and that he'd make it back to his farm outside Franklin, I turned around to face Ken Schultz.

"I've got an idea," he said, taking my arm and leading me back to my office. "I'll write up a contract for you to purchase the endocardiograph with a down payment equal to the cost of an exam—just twenty-five dollars. And I'll charge you only twenty-five dollars a month over the next eight months. By that time, Mr. Dodd should be well on his way to recovery." Ken stopped, but I knew he wasn't finished. "Okay, I'm listening," I said, smiling.

"Good, now this is the best part: You have to start out by doing regraphs weekly for two months to closely monitor his progress, and then you can regraph every other week. By charging the standard ten dollars per procedure, you'll have enough to cover your monthly payments. If you don't want to keep the machine after the eight months, you can return it without having paid a single red cent. But, I'm confident that won't be the case."

I'd already seen how valuable the endocardiograph was, and we had just used it once. I agreed to the contract and Ken left beaming.

When Mr. Dodd returned the following day, I instructed him to lie down on the adjusting table and reexamined his spine. The tender spots I found by palpating his vertebrae matched the subluxations evident on the x-rays.

I helped him sit up. "In order to restore your heart's health as much as we can," I said, "you'll have to come in for adjustments three times a week for the first month. I'll keep checking your progress with the graphs, and once we see some improvement, you can reduce your visits to twice a week—or maybe even once a week. Since the nutritional supplements have already helped, keep taking them." He nodded, wearing the same frown that had never left his face the day before. "If the regraphs show a need to change or eliminate any, we'll do it right away. I suspect you'll need less and less Phosfood as time goes on."

I let him know what to expect during an adjustment, making it clear that his vertebrae would make a popping sound as they changed position. Still, he complained, "Hey, what was that?" when he first heard the noise and remained grumpy throughout the visit.

Mr. Dodd made slow but solid progress, and we continued with the adjustments and nutritional supplements for about ten months. (By that time, the endocardiograph had a permanent place in my office, and I used it regularly for many of my patients.) He was down to a twice-a-month schedule and thankfully his demeanor had changed. I'd often found myself dreading his appointments because of his crankiness. Eventually, though, he stopped grumbling and started greeting me with a smile. I decided it was a lot easier for him to be cheerful when he was feeling well.

On one visit he asked me to look at a spot on the inside of his left thigh. I recognized it immediately as *ringworm*, a fungal infection found in the skin, hair, or nails.

"My doctor gave me some salve to rub into the area," Mr. Dodd explained, "but it didn't do any good. I thought I'd ask you about it before spending any more time and money going back to him."

"That looks like ringworm to me. I had it myself when I was in the navy, and the medical corpsman painted the area with a 4 percent iodine solution—burned like sin. Actually, it *did* burn the top layer of skin as well as the ringworm. In about three days, a paper-thin scab fell off and the ringworm was gone. I'll see if I can get some iodine, and we'll take care of it at your next appointment."

"I'm not sure I can wait that long—it itches like all get out. If you can get that stuff today, I'll be back tomorrow."

I managed to locate some iodine, and within a week the ringworm had disappeared.

Over time Mr. Dodd improved to the point that he took twenty-seven acres out of the soil bank and returned to farming on a small scale. "Just to have something to do," he told me.

Several years later, he called me on a summer morning. "I just saw Alma have a bad car accident as she turned into our driveway." His voice was shaking. "I was sitting on the front porch waiting for her to come back from grocery shopping. I called the hospital and now I'm calling you." He took a gulp of air. "My heart is pounding so hard and jumping all over the place. I'll be at your office tomorrow—God willing. Now, I've got to go and try to help her."

Heart attack victims are susceptible to having another attack if they suddenly experience some kind of trauma. I marveled at Mr. Dodd's wherewithal to call me before going to his wife's aid. He did make it to my office the next day, and a new graph showed some heart irregularities, but in general its strength was amazing. I adjusted him and gave him some additional supplements. It turned out that the incident had no impact on his overall well-being.

Mr. Dodd followed a maintenance schedule until I moved my practice to Boulder, Colorado, in 1969. I received a surprise letter from him about four years later. He gave me a brief summary of his health and activities, and described a vacation he and Alma had taken to the Finger Lakes region in upstate New York. "I wanted to visit the area where I'd grown up," he wrote. "We drove 2,943 miles in our little Ford Falcon." He told me they had moved to a retirement residence in Olivia, Minnesota, and then he came to the point of the letter: "You remember the ringworm I had on my leg, don't you? I've got it again, and both my doctor and chiropractor have no idea what you painted it with. Can you send me the information, or write to Dr. Whilhite, my chiropractor in Redwood Falls, so he can get it?"

When I first saw Leonard Dodd feebly enter my clinic, he was sixty-seven years old. Eighteen years had passed between then and the letter, making him eighty-five the last time I heard from him. As I mentioned in the previous chapter, "Someone up there looks after me." Here, again, I was given the chance to follow up on a patient several years after we had lost contact. I don't know when Leonard died, but I do believe that my chiropractic and nutritional care added many years—and fruitful years—to the life of a very ill man.

Author's Note:

In 1987, fifty years after the development of the endocardiograph, Drs. Schmidt and Goodheart began reexamining this important healing tool. Nine years later, they introduced the *acoustic cardiograph*, a more up-to-date version of Dr. Lee's design.

This device is different from the electrocardiograph, a common diagnostic instrument used by medical doctors. The electrocardiograph measures only surface electrical impulses as they move through the heart and records the information on an electrocardiogram, or EKG. Although it can reveal damaged or traumatized heart tissue, the electrocardiograph cannot provide the information on heart function or efficiency that the acoustic cardiograph can, nor can it provide a window into the body's dietary and nutritional health.

5

Our Two Babies
Prenatal Chiropractic Care

> The first duty of the obstetrician is to lessen as much as possible the amount of pain suffered in childbirth.
> *B. Frank Scholl, M.D.*
> *1926*

My four years in chiropractic college taught me that regular adjustments are especially important for an expectant mother. Flexible spine and pelvic joints as well as strong nerve flow are essential for the health of the mom, the development of the baby, and for a relatively easy delivery. I observed these benefits personally with my own wife and the birth of my two sons. This is *our* story.

Shirley and I were married June 27, 1953, and almost three years later, our first boy entered the world. Shirley's father was Carl Oscar Lilljestrale, the long-term village recorder for the Village of Clarkfield, Minnesota. My wife wanted to name our son after her father, although we decided "Carl Rude" was too short and "Oscar Rude" was too old-fashioned. We finally agreed on Carlton to honor her dad and on Grant (my middle name) as his middle name. As a result, we named our new little one Carlton Grant Lilljestrale Rude. He is now employed as a property manager in the movie industry. (And as his proud papa, I would like to brag that he handled all the props for *Sling Blade*, the Academy Award–nominated film starring Billy Bob Thornton.)

PRENATAL CARE

Throughout Shirley's pregnancy with Carlton, I made sure she had regular adjustments weekly—and sometimes twice weekly—as part of her prenatal care. When her labor contractions began on a Sunday in early May, I called the doctor and he urged us to get to the hospital immediately. We lived in Renville County, a large farming area in southwestern Minnesota with a population of about twenty thousand people. At that time only one hospital served the entire area, and it was centrally located in Olivia, fourteen miles west of our hometown of Hector. Shirley and I rushed to the car, and I sped us to the hospital.

On the way, Shirley's contractions started coming much more frequently. When we reached the hospital, we went straight to the emergency entrance. Nurses met us at the door with a wheelchair, and Shirley was whisked off to the delivery room. After parking the car, I headed for the waiting room to join the other expectant fathers. This was 1956 and dads were not allowed in the delivery room—the idea had not yet been considered. We had to agonize elsewhere, pacing the floor. I didn't have a chance to do much pacing, though, because Dr. Dahle appeared almost instantly with the news that I was the father of a healthy baby boy. The total elapsed time between calling the doctor and hearing "you're a daddy" was less than twenty-five minutes.

The odds were stacked against such an easy deliver: Carlton weighed eight pounds, twelve ounces—certainly larger than average; he was the first-born child—first deliveries tend to be the hardest; and Shirley was thirty years old—typically older first-time moms have more difficult labors. Nevertheless, the whole event passed so calmly and quickly that I barely had time to park the car.

On my way to work the next day, I stopped at the post office and bumped into Buck Nelson, a local businessman and the owner of Buck's Cafe. He chided, "Doesn't your wife know she's not supposed to labor on Sunday?"

Three and a half years later, we were expecting our second baby, due right after the beginning of the New Year, 1960. Shirley suggested we open gifts on Christmas Eve just in case the baby arrived early. She didn't want a new sibling to upstage the festivities for Carlton. Grandma and Grandpa Rude joined us to watch their wide-eyed grandson dive in and rip open his large stack of presents.

After all the gifts had been opened, we put the tired little guy to bed, and my parents left for home. Shirley and I were cleaning up the wreckage when a close friend called to invite her to the midnight service at the Methodist Church. I stayed home with a sleeping Carlton and finished putting the house back together while Shirley went off to church. She returned shortly after midnight and we went to bed.

Close to five o'clock on Christmas morning, Shirley's grunting noises woke me. "Ugh, ugh, ugh," I heard, yet she was still fast asleep.

"Is the baby coming?" I whispered, shaking her only partially awake.

"What? The baby? No, I don't think so. I'm just a little uncomfortable—probably from sitting on those hard pews. Go back to sleep."

Less than an hour later, she shook *me* awake. "The baby *is* coming," she cried. The situation had suddenly become critical. I jumped out of bed and ran down the hall, through the living room, and into the kitchen. I grabbed for the phone and called Dr. Anderson.

"I'll meet you at the hospital right away," he instructed. Knowing that second deliveries are typically easier and faster than first ones, we had no time to waste. When I ran back to the bedroom, Shirley was sitting on the edge of the bed. "We can't leave Carlton alone. Call your mother and have her come over."

I rushed back to the kitchen, called Grandma, and asked her to hurry over to babysit. Back to the bedroom again, I found Shirley close to a panic. "Better call Doc—I won't make it to the hospital!"

I ping-ponged back to the phone. Dr. Anderson was almost out the door. I heard his wife yell to him, "Go straight to their house. She's not going to make it to the hospital!" He lived only three blocks from our house so I felt relieved. When I raced back to the bedroom, I was startled to see a newborn baby lying between his mama's thighs.

Just then the doorbell rang and Dr. Anderson was on the scene. "Get some bath towels," he ordered, and I quickly obeyed. My mother came into the bedroom a few minutes later, and the doctor handed her Kirby, her brand new grandson, wrapped in a bath towel.

After the sense of urgency had passed and the commotion quieted down, Shirley explained, "I felt only three contractions: as the head came, then the shoulders, and then the rest of him. If they were all that simple, I'd have a dozen of them." And Kirby was even larger than Carlton had been, weighing an ounce more than his older brother.

Word travels fast in a small town. Later that afternoon, I went downtown and stopped into Buck's Cafe. Buck Nelson waited on me. "You know," he said, grinning, "your wife would do just about anything to get out of cooking Christmas dinner."

There is no guarantee every expectant mother who has received chiropractic prenatal care will have deliveries as smooth as Shirley's. At the same time, though, I can assure any woman that chiropractic will definitely ease the birthing process.

6

Herb's Dislocated Shoulder
Early Intervention

The public is looking for doctors who have open minds, open hearts, and a wide range of skills to help them gain and maintain their health.

Monty Wilburn, D.C.
2001 President, Colorado Chiropractic Association

Herb Johnson, one of Hector's first residents, grew up on a farm in the small rural community. In 1917 America entered World War I, and Herb enlisted in the army to fight for his country. After the armistice ended "the war to end all wars," he came back home and returned to farming. Along with other Hector veterans, he became a charter member of the Carl O. Potter Post 135 of the American Legion. Seldom missing a meeting, Herb remained a devoted member, serving as an officer at every rank. He routinely joined other legionnaires as they proudly formed the color guard in the parade on Armistice Day (officially named Veteran's Day in 1954).

At the end of World War II, soldiers returning from Germany and the South Pacific also became members of Post 135, creating a mixture of veterans now a generation apart. Within a decade, the old guard passed the leadership baton to the younger members, and a World War II vet was elected legion commander.

Upon returning from my own tour of duty in the navy, I also joined the Carl O. Potter Post. I must confess I wasn't as zealous as

Herb and didn't regularly attend the meetings, although ultimately I did serve as post commander for two years.

Near the end of his first term in office, President Eisenhower read a report stating that American youth had scored lower than European children in a battery of physical fitness tests. Responding to these dismal results, the president established the President's Council on Youth Fitness in 1956 to encourage children to lead healthy and active lives.

Causing quite a stir in the media, this report was featured as the top news story for three or four days. Marvin Shiro, the post commander, brought a Minneapolis newspaper to the monthly meeting. Pointing to the front page articles, he said, "The papers are full of stuff about American youth's deplorable shape, and we need to do something about it. I say we set an example for them. C'mon, everybody stand up."

Marvin led the group of old and new vets in well-known military calisthenics. "Now, let's do some push-ups," he ordered.

A dance had been held the night before at the legion club and the floor still had not been swept. Some small beads of dance wax littered the area where the vets were exercising. Not wanting to get his hands dirty, Herb stepped into the men's room to get a few paper towels. He had already vigorously participated in the "windmill" and jumping jacks, and he was ready to put his all into push-ups. He refused to be outdone by any of those "young whippersnappers."

As Herb placed his hands on the paper towels and lifted his body for the push-up, one hand slipped sideways on the waxed floor, and he collapsed in pain—he'd dislocated his shoulder.

The meeting came to an abrupt halt. Someone immediately called the local physician, whose wife expressed regret that her husband was out of town attending a convention. "Hey, maybe we should call Dr. Rude," a legionnaire shouted above the crowd. "Chiropractors work on joints, so he probably knows how to take care of a dislocated shoulder."

When I received the emergency call at home, I told them to meet me at my office in fifteen minutes.

Herb's dislocated shoulder was actually the first of its kind I'd ever treated. At that time, I was enrolled in a three-year postgraduate course at Northwestern College of Chiropractic leading to certification as a Diplomate in Chiropractic Orthopedics (DABCO). And just two weeks earlier, we had studied all the possible problems in and around the shoulder, but I hadn't as yet reset one.

I carefully examined Herb's injury. The head of the right *humerus* (the large bone in the upper arm) hung low—in front of the rib cage—and his arm drooped at a precarious angle. He held his right elbow with his left hand, trying to support the injured arm. I took an x-ray to see precisely how the head of the humerus had shifted.

After studying the x-ray, I reviewed my notes to determine what protocol to follow because a shoulder can dislocate in different directions depending on the mechanism of injury. I performed a *Kocher maneuver* (essentially applying downward pressure on the humerus while gently rotating the arm) and guided the head of the humerus back into place on the first try. Then I taped the shoulder to prevent it from slipping out again. After making a sling to support the weight of the arm, I recommended he go home and pack his shoulder in ice. (Ice reduces the swelling and helps to contract the overstretched ligaments.)

To monitor his condition closely, I instructed Herb to return the next morning, at which time I reexamined him. "Your shoulder tissues are torn," I explained, "and during the normal healing process, a lot of scar tissue is usually formed. You could develop a frozen shoulder, preventing you from having full use of your arm, unless we take steps to keep that from happening."

I showed him two exercises that would help minimize scar tissue formation: First, while he stood slightly bent forward at the waist, I directed him to let his arm hang and make small circular movements, encouraging him to gradually widen the circle as healing occurred. Second, I told him to closely face a wall and gently walk his fingers up and down it, increasing his range of motion as he improved. I cautioned Herb to start slowly and exercise only to the point of pain.

We also discussed using *diathermy* on his shoulder in a day or two. This form of physical therapy involves the application of electromagnetic energy to an affected area. The resistance of the body tissue to the flow of this energy produces heat, speeding up circulation and therefore the rate of healing. I chose to wait two to three days in case the blood vessels in Herb's shoulder had been damaged. Using diathermy too soon could have increased the risk of hemorrhage.

Herb was a good patient, meticulously following my instructions. His shoulder healed completely, free of any restriction or pain, and his full normal range of motion returned. At his final checkup, he asked, "Can I send in a claim to my insurance company for this?"

His question surprised me. After all, this was 1956, and insurance companies did *not* pay chiropractic claims. "You know, Herb, it's highly unlikely they'll pay, but I'll send it in for you anyway. Maybe it'll jar them into realizing that policyholders go to chiropractors too."

When I filed the claim, I included a detailed explanation for each charge: the exam, the x-ray, the resetting of the shoulder, and the multiple diathermy treatments. The fees totaled ninety dollars. (Now, nearly fifty years later, I realize I had forgotten to charge for taping his shoulder. . . .)

A short while later, I received a check for the entire amount along with a letter stating, "We are pleased to pay this claim. Our policyholder probably received better care at your hands than he would have at any other medical facility." It was signed by the medical director of the insurance company.

Much has changed over the last half century. Fortunately, because of extensive postgraduate education, many twenty-first century chiropractors are now able to treat conditions far beyond the scope of the typical back injury. In addition, over the past fifty years, insurance companies have made a huge shift in their policies and are now paying for chiropractic services. Unfortunately, however, these same companies have changed their attitude toward policyholders. In 1956, the medical director was most concerned about the care rendered to the *policyholder*. Today, profits for the *shareholder* seem to matter the most, often at the expense of quality medical care.

7

The Story of Gigi
Chiropractic for Animals

> If you have a health problem caused by a spinal misalignment, you can take all the medication in the world and it may cover up your symptoms, but only a chiropractic adjustment will fix it permanently.
>
> *Donald Zisch, D.C.*
> *First President, Colorado State Chiropractic Society*

Throughout our years in Minnesota, Shirley and I frequently socialized with our close friends Barbara and Don. We knew they longed to have children, and although Barb had been pregnant several times, she spontaneously miscarried in her first or second trimester. These miscarriages had taken such a heavy toll on both of them that they decided to adopt a child. In the meantime, during the long and tedious adoption process, Barb lavished motherly affection on Gigi, her adorable poodle puppy. She doted upon this little white ball of fur, giving her a shampoo and rinse every week, painting her toenails, and tying ribbons in her hair. Gigi was her surrogate baby.

Barb and Don agreed that moving from their second-floor apartment to a larger, new home might facilitate the adoption. Since Don was the local veterinarian with a substantial practice caring for all the farm animals in the Hector area, they could easily afford a lot on a quiet cul-de-sac in a new development. The lengthy adoption process allowed adequate time for the completion of the construction.

For a small rural town of roughly one thousand people, their beautiful two-story house was quite a showplace, a "Parade of Homes." It boasted a winding cobblestone walkway, retractable awnings, a large living-room fireplace, and sliding glass doors leading from the dining room to a spacious patio and backyard. Also, in keeping with the decorating trends of the late 1960s, the entire ground floor was carpeted in white shag. But most noteworthy was the home's unique heating system: special, factory-ordered electric panels wired right into the drywall. This feature attracted curious people from miles around eager to see if such an innovation could withstand Minnesota winters.

By the time they moved into their new home, Gigi was housebroken and nearly a full-sized poodle. When she scratched at the glass door in the dining room, Barb and Don knew she needed to go outside, and they allowed her to roam throughout the neighborhood.

Despite the low traffic in their cul-de-sac, one evening a car accidentally struck Gigi. Luckily she lived, with no broken bones and just a few abrasions. Sadly, though, the impact did significantly paralyze her hind quarters. Unable to stand on all fours, Gigi had to drag herself around by her front legs, and she lost control of her bladder and bowels as well. Even though Don administered the best care veterinarian medicine could offer, he couldn't reverse the paralysis. The pristine white carpeting was starting to take a beating.

After a week of cleaning up after Gigi's accidents, Don had to admit that putting their poodle to sleep was the best solution. As far as Barb was concerned, however, this was tantamount to murder. "You can't kill my baby!" she cried.

Barbara insisted on trying something else. She called us on a Saturday morning and asked Shirley, "Do you suppose Kenn would take a look at Gigi? I waited until today to call because I didn't think he'd want me to bring a dog into the office while his patients were there."

Shirley passed the phone to me. "What's the matter?" I asked.

On the verge of tears, Barb described the events of the last several days and then broke down in sobs when she reached the part about mercy killing. Maybe it was the desperate tone in her voice, maybe it was my curiosity about chiropractic adjustments for animals, or maybe it was just my tenderhearted nature, but I agreed to give it a try. "Bring her in," I told her. "I'll be there in ten minutes."

I met Don and Gigi at my office, and we sat down to discuss the problem. Although Don was much more of an authority on animal care than I, spinal mechanics is not included in the curriculum of either medical or veterinarian colleges. Not knowing how Gigi would respond to a chiropractic adjustment worried me the most. While manipulating her spine, I might damage her spinal cord and worsen her condition—she could even die. I wanted to avoid being held responsible and having a lawsuit on my hands. Don sympathized, since he faced the same risk when treating farmers' livestock. He assured me a sort of unwritten law existed protecting a doctor who did his best to help an injured animal.

I examined Gigi. Using my fingers, I palpated her back and felt a spot where the *spinous processes* (bony protrusions) of the vertebrae were badly misaligned—approximately at the level of the human T9, the ninth thoracic vertebra. I suggested we x-ray her back, although I wasn't sure how I'd set up the x-ray machine for a small dog. I reasoned that Gigi's trunk was nearly the size of a man's neck. I measured her body and looked up the proper settings for filming a man's neck matching that size. My idea worked perfectly, and after developing the film, I clearly saw the cause of her problem: a precise subluxation between T10 and T11—the eleventh thoracic vertebra had shifted forward in relation to the tenth.

When I showed the x-ray to Don, he hesitated briefly and then said, "Okay, let's get on with it and see what happens."

I positioned Gigi over the small stool where I normally sit while palpating a patient's neck. Her front legs were on one side of the square top, and her hind legs hung limply down on the other. This cushioned area appeared to be an adequate surface for a reasonable adjustment. I then palpated Gigi's spine and placed my hands at the subluxation.

"Kneel down and raise her head," I told Don, "so she won't have to hold it up by contracting her back muscles." He did as I instructed. I made a short, sharp thrust, and we both heard a loud pop, just as if I'd adjusted a human. Gigi made no reaction—she didn't whine, bark, or show any sign of pain or fear. She remained still, without changing her position.

When I lifted her off the stool and placed her on the floor, she stood upright on all four legs. I went to the door and called her, and she started to walk, following me as I proceeded through the front door and then outside. Don and I watched as she easily maneuvered the three small steps, walked onto the grassy yard, squatted, and relieved herself. She began running and jumping, and then she rolled in the grass as if the accident had never happened. We were stunned. Chiropractic had come to the rescue again, saving a pet from euthanasia and sparing its owner heartbreak.

Chiropractic obviously works just as well for animals as it does for people—not surprising, as all mammals have similar spinal anatomy. I know of several veterinarians who studied chiropractic and have now integrated it into their practice. Dr. Ralph Wiggins, D.C., a good friend of mine, was interested in learning how to care for his treasured quarter horses with chiropractic. He took a postgraduate course from a doctor who is a vet as well as a chiropractor. Since then he has adjusted large and small animals, from horses to gerbils, and he claims that horses are easier to adjust than people. I have heard that a number of professional race-horse breeders employ chiropractic-trained vets for their prize-winning racing steeds.

Without a doubt, chiropractic is extremely effective—for both man *and* beast.

8

Barb's Babies
A Remedy for Miscarriage

> Man is a reasoning animal
> *Seneca*

Barb shouted with joy when she saw her poodle's miraculous recovery. Gigi's ordeal had introduced her to the power of chiropractic, prompting Barb to seriously consider her own health. Quite unique for Americans at that time, she believed strongly in the benefits of daily meditation. One morning while deep in thought, she wondered suddenly, "If a misalignment in Gigi's spine caused her to lose control of her bladder and bowels, is it possible I have a misalignment that's preventing me from carrying a pregnancy to full term?" The search for an answer brought Barb to my office.

Suspecting a female doctor might make her more comfortable, I included my mother, Beatrice Rude, D.C., in the consultation. After Barb described her medical history, we assured her that a *subluxation complex* (several misaligned vertebrae) in her pelvis or lower spine was probably connected to her miscarriages during the first or second trimester.

My mother went on to explain that we might actually find a minor misalignment that was changing into a major one when her fetus reached a certain size. "You see," she said, "the lower back is the area where the nerves to the reproductive organs branch off from the spinal cord and pass through openings between the vertebrae. A non-pregnant woman has a normal amount of swayback curvature in her lower back, but that changes during pregnancy. As the fetus grows, the mom becomes more swaybacked to compensate for the added bulk and weight. When the baby develops enough to force a change in posture, a slight subluxation becomes a lot more pronounced, substantially narrowing those nerve openings. This can lead to a reduction in the vital nerve flow to the pelvic region, definitely increasing the chances of miscarriage."

"Okay, that sounds reasonable," Barb said. "So how do we figure out what's wrong?"

To provide her with an accurate diagnosis, we recommended a thorough chiropractic examination and follow-up x-rays. "Is there any possibility you're pregnant now?" I asked. She shook her head no. I pointed out that it's inadvisable to x-ray a pregnant woman unless absolutely necessary because of the potential radiation risk to the unborn baby.

My mother and I performed the physical exam. While Barb lay face down on the adjusting table, we palpated each vertebra, checking for tenderness or an abnormal position that would indicate a subluxation. We focused especially on the nerves associated with the female reproductive system in the lower back.

"This area right here," I said, pressing on the lowest vertebra, "is L5. Radiating out from this spot is the fifth lumbar nerve, which supplies most of the nerve flow to the uterus."

Barb jerked away from my fingers. "Gee, that's really sore."

"That's what we'd expect from your history," I said. "Now, let's move up your spine." As soon as I reached L3, two vertebrae above L5, and pressed down, Barb twisted in pain. "Again, not surprising," I told her. "The third lumbar nerve leaves the spinal cord at this level—it's responsible for supplying the ovaries."

To confirm both L3 and L5 were out of alignment, we tested the strength of specific muscles that share the same nerve supply as Barb's reproductive organs. This technique is based on the knowledge that each spinal nerve has three branches: *sensory*, *motor*, and *visceral*. The sensory branch begins in the skin and carries messages from the environment to the brain (touch, temperature, and pain); the motor branch communicates with the muscles; and the visceral branch, the internal organs. A misalignment involving a spinal nerve can affect one, two, or all three branches. Checking for muscle weakness is a simple way to gather more clues about a subluxation at any level of the spine.

The *gluteus medius* muscle (located outside the hip bone) shares the ovary nerve supply, and the *gluteus maximus* muscle (the large buttocks muscle) shares the uterine nerve supply. Barb's muscles showed extreme weakness on both the right and left sides, supporting our initial findings.

Spinal percussion, still another technique for verifying joint abnormalities, is best explained in the textbook *Musculoskeletal Pain: Diagnosis and Physical Treatment.** This method involves tapping each vertebra with a reflex hammer and evaluating the patient's pain: For basic subluxations, the patient will feel a sharp pain that quickly dissipates; for disease conditions, the pain will be deep and throbbing, lasting a short time; and for a slipped disk in the lower back, the brief, sharp pain will also be present in the leg.

When we tapped Barb's L3 and L5 vertebrae, she described a short, intense pain at both levels without leg discomfort—further evidence of spinal misalignments.

The x-rays supported our diagnosis. "Barb, all the results agree," I said. "The joints between the affected vertebrae are not functioning correctly, which compromises the nerves coming out of your spine at those levels. This faulty nerve function relates directly to your reproductive organs."

"Well, can you fix me like you fixed Gigi?"

My mother nodded. "There's a good possibility of that. Let's start with a treatment plan of frequent chiropractic adjustments and *intersegmental traction*—that's a form of physical therapy that increases stability and flexibility of the spine."

Barb came to us three times a week for the first five weeks, tapering off to twice weekly for the next two months and then finally to once a week. "I never realized my lower back was so stiff," she told us. "I thought it was normal. Now, after coming here for a while, I can move much more freely than I used to."

During the eighteenth week of care, Barb came in looking excited. "I missed my period last week," she said. "I must be pregnant." An examination by her medical doctor confirmed the news. She

---

*David A. Zohn, M.D., and John McM. Mennell, M.D., *Musculoskeletal Pain: Diagnosis and Physical Treatment* (Boston: Little, Brown and Company, 1976), p. 61.

continued her weekly adjustments, and as each week passed without difficulty or the threat of miscarriage, Barb became more ecstatic. "This pregnancy has lasted longer than all the others!" she exclaimed when she entered her third and last trimester. Everything appeared to be progressing normally.

Barb persisted with her weekly appointments. Near her due date, she delivered a perfectly healthy baby boy. Her delight and preoccupation with her new son took up most of her time, and she stopped visiting our office.

Twenty-one months later, another baby boy joined the household. The pregnancy passed smoothly without the risk of miscarriage, yet the delivery was more difficult than the first—contrary to what typically occurs. Barb turned to meditation for guidance and then came to see me.

"Was Billy's delivery harder than Jimmy's because I didn't have any adjustments for almost two years?"

"Yes, I'm sure," I said. "Chiropractic care most definitely would have eased his birth." Consequently, she returned to having spinal adjustments on a regular basis. "I just feel better all over when your mother works on my back," she told me one day after her appointment.

A few years later, Barb and Don had a daughter, followed by a third son three years after that. All four children were delivered normally without complications, and today they are adults. Both Jimmy and Billy married, and they have at least seven children between them. I lost track of the family tree when I moved to Colorado, but most likely the other two children have married as well.

The story doesn't end there. In a small town like Hector, Minnesota, everyone knows almost everything about everyone else. When word of Barb's normal pregnancies spread, especially after her many miscarriages, other women with similar problems visited my office. Donna became a patient and soon delivered a baby girl, followed by a baby boy, without a hitch. Another woman, Clarisse, had a fifteen-year-old son but had not been able to carry any subsequent pregnancies to term. After hearing about Barb's success, she came to the Rude Center for spinal adjustments. Her history showed she had fallen down a flight of stairs when her son was about two years old. This undoubtedly led to the subluxation in her lower back. Within eight months of treatment, Clarisse conceived and ultimately delivered a healthy baby girl.

It gives me tremendous satisfaction to know that chiropractic was responsible for the birth of more than a dozen children and grandchildren. And to think it all started with a little white poodle who went wandering one evening.

9

Dr. Roush's Comments
Not a Placebo

> What Americans call alternative medicine is traditional healing in 80 percent of the world.
> *Donald M. Peterson Jr.*
> *Editor and Publisher,* Dynamic Chiropractor

Toward the late 1960s, a few years after Gigi's dramatic healing success, I traveled from Minnesota to Kansas City for a chiropractic seminar. One of the scheduled lecturers was the renowned Dr. Clarence Gonstead, the developer of the Gonstead Technique.* A licensed pilot, he was flying his own plane from Wisconsin to Kansas City. Unfortunately, he had to make an emergency landing en route and telephoned to explain he'd be late. After apologizing to the attendees, the convention chairman said, "So I guess you'll have a free hour to do as you please. I hope we won't lose too many of you in the bar."

As the audience started to leave, one doctor in the front row shouted above the noise, "I'd like to make a suggestion." All of us turned to him and after we quieted down, he continued, "I'm sure every doctor here has truly phenomenal experiences with some patients who respond to treatments better and faster than expected. We

---

*One of the many methods used to analyze and adjust the spine, this technique is part of the curriculum at some, but not all, of the seventeen chiropractic colleges in the United States.

get a thrill from those results. And then we have the run-of-the-mill variety, the patients who improve on schedule, just as anticipated. The slow-to-recover cases are gratifying, though not quite as exciting. But then there are the rare situations—the extremely troubling ones—when we do all that we can and the patient simply makes no progress. Frankly, during those times, I get depressed. I feel like I haven't fulfilled my oath as a Doctor of Chiropractic, and it gnaws at me. I become disheartened and remain that way for several days, feeling responsible for letting down the patient."

I didn't know the distinguished-looking gentleman who had made such an impassioned speech. Everyone's eyes and ears focused on him, tuned in to his words. No one uttered a sound. I learned later that he was Dr. Bill Roush of Pueblo, Colorado, a 1938 graduate of the Palmer School of Chiropractic. He was a member of the Board of Regents of the New York College of Chiropractic.

"I propose we stay here," he said, "and take turns describing our most extraordinary patients. In that way, we can renew our enthusiasm and faith in our chosen profession. When we return to our offices on Monday morning, it will be with our passion restored." He paused, waiting for a response.

Nearly all of the attending doctors agreed with his idea and returned to their seats. Dr. Roush was the first to speak about a patient who had suffered from a malfunctioning gall bladder. When he finished, he pointed to the doctor on the far side of the first row to continue. As each one stood and provided an example of successful chiropractic care, we heard about a host of ailments that chiropractors treat: sinus problems, chronic sacroiliac, headaches, slipped disks, infant colic, premenstrual syndrome, fibromyalgia, tonsillitis, bed-wetting, asthma, high blood pressure, constipation, *thoracic outlet syndrome* (pain radiating down the arm), carpal tunnel, vertigo, and many more. Most of the participants emphasized that the patient had chosen chiropractic as a last resort. Everyone seemed determined to avoid repeating a health condition; nevertheless, about halfway through the crowd, we started hearing second iterations, which merely reinforced what had already been said.

I wanted to share something unique, though that was going to be difficult since I was seated in the back row and would be the third from the last to speak. My six-year-old patient with a leaking heart valve came to mind, but just then a doctor about seven people ahead of me described a very similar case.

Suddenly, I remembered Gigi—no one had discussed adjusting an animal. So I presented her story, and as I was finishing, ending with, "She walked onto the grassy yard, squatted, and relieved herself," Dr. Roush rose to his feet and again interrupted the proceedings.

"I'd like to thank you for that remarkable discourse. You just did three things: First, you proved that spinal misalignments can impair internal organs. Second, you may have triggered new thoughts about chiropractic for pets. And third—by far the most important—you did something you probably didn't realize. Throughout the years, the medical profession has more or less equated chiropractic with faith healing. The fantastic results from spinal adjustments have been shrugged off as stemming from a placebo effect. M.D.'s don't understand our work and have inferred that a chiropractor succeeds because the patient expects to recover. Your small poodle had no idea what your goal was when you adjusted her. It wasn't a question of her having faith in you or faith in chiropractic. She didn't expect a miracle cure, yet she was totally healed, wasn't she?"

His astute observation and forthright manner impressed me. When it was convenient, I introduced myself and thanked him for leading the group in such a valuable exercise. After my move to Boulder, Colorado, we became good friends.

Thanks to Dr. Roush, when I went to work the Monday morning after the conference, I did feel reenergized—he had certainly helped rekindle my devotion. His profound message had further strengthened my belief in the potent healing science we call chiropractic.

10

A Flower Child
From Sinus Infection to Diarrhea

> It's supposed to be a secret, but I will tell you anyway. We doctors do nothing. We only help and encourage the doctor within.
>
> *Dr. Albert Schweitzer*

In the late 1960s and early 1970s "flower children" roamed all over the nation, and Boulder, Colorado, was their Mecca. Traveling in old beat-up Volkswagen vans covered in psychedelic paint, they were attracted to this area like flies to honey. The comfortable summer months and the many opportunities available for camping and communing with nature were ideal for the hippie generation. The mountains just west of town are especially beautiful at that time of year, and the valleys abound with color.

When I moved to Boulder in December 1969, I contacted a realtor, who expressed concern about the invasion of these "undesirables" and their negative impact on the real estate market. He was attempting to organize a vigilante posse to "meet them at the city limits and escort them right through town so they'll know they're unwelcome in Boulder." Many of the city's well-established residents deeply resented their parks overrun with "long-haired vagrants" and their easy-going manner.

Yet sometimes we hurry to criticize the unfamiliar. My own encounters with the young people at that time were rarely disagreeable. In fact, in the summer of 1970, I had the pleasure of meeting Mary, a flower child from an affluent east-coast family. After completing her first year at Vassar, she had joined the throng of hippies descending upon Boulder. Mary's mother had always advocated chiropractic, taking her children to their chiropractor in Virginia for any health problem. Consequently, when Mary came down with a headache and sore throat, she paid me a visit.

During the initial consultation, I asked, "When did you go to a chiropractor for the first time?"

"Well, you know, I don't remember for sure," she said. "Maybe when I was two or three. We went to the chiropractor for everything—my mom insisted. And none of us ever got really sick and had to miss school." For Mary and her family, the chiropractor was their primary doctor.

Because she was also complaining about a runny nose and nasal congestion, I told her I wanted to *transilluminate* (direct a powerful light through) her sinus cavities. This procedure, performed in total darkness, detects the presence and magnitude of congestion. I used my *otoscope* (an instrument for looking into the ears) but replaced the ordinary head with a small probe that produces a strong pinpoint of light. I closed the door and turned off the overhead light.

Placing the probe into the little pocket above Mary's eyeball right next to her nose, I transilluminated her frontal sinuses. Within the skull bone, these cavities are hollow. If they're not congested, the light will shine through and onto the forehead tissue above the eye. Mary's forehead remained dark, indicating blockage was present.

Next, I checked her *maxillary* (upper jaw) sinuses. I positioned the probe just below the eyeball and directed her to tilt her head back and open her mouth as wide as possible. Without congestion, the roof of the mouth should light up like a Christmas tree. Not so for Mary. Again, I saw only darkness—additional evidence that she was suffering from severe sinus inflammation, or *sinusitis*.

"Mary, there's probably some underlying cause for your condition—it probably didn't begin on its own. Let's see what x-rays of your neck can tell us." After taking and reviewing the x-rays, I told her I saw a rather extreme misalignment of the *atlas* (the top neck vertebra) and the *condyles* (rounded nodules) of the base of the skull.

"How did I get something like that?" she asked.

"Barring a traumatic blow to the head or a whiplash type of accident, I can only guess you've been lying on the hard ground in a sleeping bag without adequate support for your neck."

She grinned, confirming I'd hit the nail on the head. "I have to admit the ground is nothing like my bed at home," she said.

I prescribed a three-part treatment: First, to relieve her sore throat pain, I placed *Wonder Oil* (see chapter 1) on a cotton swab and dabbed the back of her throat and the lower portion of her *nasopharnyx* (the nasal passages above the throat).

Second, to eliminate Mary's sinus inflammation and congestion, I used *galvanic electrotherapy*, a highly successful electrical treatment. A galvanic instrument generates a low-voltage direct current that promotes healing when introduced into the body. Applying a negative current can eliminate scar tissue, whereas a positive current can help reduce swelling, decrease nerve irritability, relieve acute pain, stop hemorrhaging—and decongest the sinuses. For that reason, when I applied the positive galvanism to Mary's forehead, her sinuses began to drain. She felt relief almost immediately.

(Electrotherapy comes in many forms and produces outstanding results, but it does require the presence of a technician during the entire treatment. Because insurance companies insist a patient be seen in the least amount of time possible, they have been reluctant to pay for this therapy, forcing most doctors to discontinue its use.)

The third part of the protocol was the most important: a series of weekly adjustments to remove the *source* of her sinus trouble. "Your symptoms will return," I cautioned, "unless we correct the subluxations in your neck." I adjusted the badly aligned vertebrae, and she made an appointment for the following week.

Our friendship grew throughout the summer as Mary regularly visited me. In late July she announced that she and three friends had decided to spend a few weeks "bumming around" in Mexico. They planned to drive their old VW van to El Paso, cross the Rio Grande into Mexico, move south across the Continental Divide, and stop in Mazatlan. On the return trip they'd travel north through Arizona and back to Colorado.

"Where are you going to sleep, and how do you plan to eat along the way?" I asked, having a good idea what her answer would be.

"Oh, we'll take our sleeping bags and just camp out under the stars most of the time. As far as eating goes, we'll probably do a lot of our own cooking. I'm sure there'll be small towns along the way where we can buy supplies. We'll be sort of roughing it."

Even though I admired her devil-may-care attitude, I had to warn Mary and her friends about the risks they'd be taking. "I'm sure you've heard about Montezuma's Revenge?" I asked. "Most of Mexico's water supply is unsanitary and untreated, especially in the sparsely populated areas. If you drink the water, you'll probably come down with a severe case of diarrhea."

"Yeah, maybe I've heard something about that...."

"Let me suggest a possible lifesaver: One of the sales reps for Standard Process Laboratories recommends their product *betaine hydrochloride* for preventing traveler's diarrhea. Although I've never visited Mexico and can't speak firsthand about their product, I have heard good things about it. It's a digestive aid that increases the acidity of the stomach enough to kill off most troublesome bugs. You have to take a tablet every time you put something in your mouth, whether it's food, water, toothbrush—anything. As long as you don't take extremely large doses, you'll have no discomfort. Simply follow my instructions, and you'll do fine."

"Sounds good to me," she said. "I'll take some along. You better give me two bottles. I don't know exactly how long we'll be gone or when we'll be coming back."

When she did return to my office six weeks later, Mary bubbled over with good news. "That stuff you gave me really worked," she said. "I didn't get the runs once during our trip. All my friends came down with it, though. I offered them some of my pills, but they refused. Brad was afraid to try them because he'd learned in chemistry that hydrochloride was an acid. I told him they wouldn't hurt him, but he ignored me. He ended up scaring Angel and Lenny so they wouldn't touch them either, which was dumb. They were miserable, and I had fun the whole time."

I thoroughly enjoyed Mary's undaunted spirit. When the weather turned cold, she migrated with her fellow hippies to warmer places, and I never saw her again. I missed her.

Unlike her friends, Mary embraced more than just conventional medicine, affording her a wider selection of healing options. Frequently, chiropractic and other alternative therapies can offer safer, more successful solutions than Western treatments. Natural substances, such as vitamins, minerals, amino acids, and herbs, are often just as effective as pharmaceuticals, yet without the harmful side effects. Trained professionals are available to educate the public about nontraditional remedies, thereby lifting the fear and mistrust that sometimes accompanies the unknown. Being open-minded and informed increases the likelihood of maintaining exceptional health.

11

An Unusual Shoulder Problem
Flat Feet

> Postural imbalances resulting from an underlying foot dysfunction often mean a patient should receive both appropriate chiropractic adjustments and long-term supportive therapy.
> *Monte Greenwalt, D.C.*
> *Founder, Foot Levelers*

When I saw Peter for the first time, my instincts warned me that he might be a challenge. A well-dressed man in his early thirties, he marched into my office, thrust out his chest, and strutted about the room. His tight clothing showed off a sculpted physique that undoubtedly resulted from extensive workouts. "I hate to say this," he said, sitting down opposite me, "especially since I've always considered myself to be in superb physical shape, but I have this sharp pain behind my left shoulder blade. It feels like someone is stabbing me with a knife."

"You know, that kind of pain could indicate a heart problem," I said. "Where is it exactly—strictly in the shoulder blade or does it also extend to the front part of the shoulder, or possibly down the inside of the upper arm?"

"Not in my arm at all and hardly in the front," he snapped. "It hurts mostly in the back between the ribs."

"How long have you had it?"

"A couple of weeks. I thought I'd just pulled a muscle during my workout so I had a massage. It helped some—still feel the pain, though. I think something in my back is out of place. That's *why* I took the time to come here." Peter tapped his foot impatiently.

"Does working out worsen the pain?" I tried to ignore his surly behavior.

"Not really. I did try extra weights and exercise to see if that would help, but it didn't, so I decided to just tough it out—except the pain is too distracting. If I don't exercise, I feel only slightly better. But there's no way I'll stop my training program—I just *have* to stay in shape."

"I'm sure I can help, but I'll need more information to pinpoint the cause of your problem. It could be a pulled *intercostal* muscle—between the ribs—or it could be a pinched nerve between two vertebrae. It's possible you have referred pain from some other injured part in the body. Let's see what an examination will tell me."

Peter gripped the sides of the chair. "How much will this cost me?" He leaned forward, his eyes narrowing.

"Well, the exam is twenty-five dollars, but x-rays may be necessary."

He lunged out of his seat. "And what will *that* cost me?" he growled, inches from my face.

I'd had enough. His blustering had finally rankled me, pushing me to become more outspoken than usual. "Look, you obviously spend a great deal on your appearance," I said, pointing my finger at him. "A designer wardrobe, gym memberships, and there are the muscle-building nutritional supplements you've listed on your intake forms. I'll bet you even drive a sports car. And you're *annoyed* about paying a relatively small amount of money to find the reason for your pain?"

My bluntness did the trick. Peter immediately calmed down and sat back in the chair. "Yeah, you're right," he mumbled. "My body *is* my most prized possession, and maybe I shouldn't skimp on fixing it." He managed a thin smile.

I examined him and he did appear to have a pinched nerve. The x-rays confirmed my diagnosis. I explained the results to Peter and then began the treatment for resolving his pain: First, after instructing him to lie face down on the adjusting table, I checked his entire spine by palpating each vertebra. When I touched the misaligned vertebrae, Peter tensed his back muscles and complained about some discomfort. I adjusted all but the thoracic subluxations by applying pressure on the vertebrae, "freeing" them to align properly.

"Now, for the second part," I said. "I need to adjust the middle of your back a little differently. Turn over, sit up, and lock your hands behind your neck. Next, put your elbows together and bend over until your elbows are touching your navel." With Peter coiled in this position, I wrapped my arms around him, rolled him back onto the table and adjusted his back with a thrust to the thoracic vertebrae—an *anterior thoracic move*. His vertebrae bounced back into place and his spine realigned.

"Wow, that felt great!" His face brightened. "The pain is almost completely gone. So quick and easy. It's a miracle."

I let him know there'd be some temporary residual soreness that would eventually subside. He scheduled a checkup for the next day. Relaxed now, he was clearly a changed man as he left the office, looking pleased he'd come to see me.

"I feel terrific," Peter told me the following afternoon. "I'm not sure I even need to be here." Nevertheless, I examined him and identified only two tender areas in his spine that needed adjusting. Oddly enough, the anterior thoracic problem had not reappeared.

On Monday, however, Peter was back in my office. "The stabbing pain is back again," he grumbled. "I was doing just fine through Saturday, and then during my run on Sunday, I started hurting after about two miles. It isn't as bad as the first time, but it's still there."

"I'll just check you all over again."

"I was in such great shape for three days. What's going on?"

I wasn't exactly sure. In the treatment room, I examined his back and repeated the same treatment from his first visit, including the anterior thoracic move. Sitting up with a smile, Peter said, "The pain is gone. You fixed it again."

He scheduled an appointment to return on Wednesday, although later he canceled because he was feeling so good.

Not for long. On the following Monday, Peter returned to my office. "I started hurting again on Sunday during my run," he said. Again, I adjusted him, repeating the anterior thoracic move, and he went to work relieved.

Yet on the following Monday, he was back *again*. "I don't understand it—the pain seems to begin every week while I'm running. I run only once a week to keep my legs in shape. Otherwise, I exercise at the gym. Lots of people run and they don't have this problem. What am I doing wrong?"

Voilà! It finally dawned on me—*his feet*! Because I hadn't asked Peter to remove his shoes during the initial exam, I hadn't studied his feet. I asked him now to take off his shoes and pants, and stand facing me.

Immediately, I could see he had foot *pronation*, also known as flat feet or fallen arches—one of the most common foot problems. I looked at five different areas to confirm my diagnosis (anyone can check these at home):

1. *Patella (kneecap) position.* I examined Peter's knees as he stood directly in front of me. I told him to relax and look straight ahead. Normally the patellae point forward, but Peter's knee caps rotated inward, as if they were trying to face each other.

2. *Foot position.* I instructed Peter to step out into the hall and walk toward me. As he moved, I saw his toes point outward rather than straight ahead—an abnormal condition known as *foot flare*.

3. *Achilles tendon.* I told him to turn around and walk away from me, so I could observe his legs and feet from the rear. The Achilles tendon should extend from the calf muscle of the leg straight down to the heel bone, or *calcaneus*. Peter's tendons, though, had a definite curvature toward the outside—another indicator of fallen arches.

4. *Shoe wear.* I checked the heels of his shoes and found excessive wear on the outside—a sure sign of pronation.

5. *Arch space.* While Peter remained standing, I knelt down and tried to slip my fingers under the arch of each foot. In this position, there is normally enough room for two fingers to fit up to their first knuckle. In Peter's case, there was absolutely no room under his arches.

Without question, he had fallen arches and was an ideal candidate for arch correction.

My experience told me that pronation also put Peter's *psoas muscles* at a mechanical disadvantage. These muscles run from the inside of the *femur* (thigh bone) up through the bottom of the pelvis and fasten onto the five lumbar vertebrae in the lower back. With Peter lying face up on the exam table, I tested the strength of each muscle: I held his leg slightly outward and above the table, and directed him to hold the position while I tried to push his leg down and out, thus stressing the psoas muscle. Under normal circumstances, a patient should be able to resist this pressure. But, just as I had expected, the muscles on both of Peter's legs exhibited considerable weakness.

To verify this finding was due to his flat feet, I devised a makeshift method for providing arch support: I tore off two pieces of two-inch-wide adhesive tape, each about thirty inches long. I stuck the center of one piece underneath his right foot. With one half of the tape, I wrapped the inside of his foot, pulled up on his arch, crossed over the instep, and affixed the end to the *outside* of his lower calf. With the other half, I wrapped the outside of his foot, brought it across the instep, and attached the end to the *inside* of the lower leg. This strapping elevated the arch to some degree. I did the same for the left foot. Then I retested the psoas muscles and found them to be stronger.

"That tape makes a *huge* difference," he said.

"I think I've figured out why your pain comes back every time you go running on Sunday."

"Great! I knew there had to be something wrong." He sat up and faced me. "What is it? I want to get rid of it."

"You have foot pronation caused by severe fallen arches," I explained. "Because adjusting your back relieves the shoulder pain, I'm certain the chiropractic treatment is correct up to that point. But the problem obviously returns when you run. Running jars the spine and causes the adjustment to slip because there's something unstable—specifically, your flat feet and resulting weak psoas muscles. They make it difficult for the body to handle the pounding on the pavement, forcing it into a counterbalancing act. You see, the body is a wonderful machine. It will always try to minimize one problem by shifting itself, although that may lead to new symptoms—like your shoulder pain. You could see that after I taped the arch, the muscles tested stronger. *Orthotics*, or arch supports, are definitely the answer."

"Oh, I've known for years I have flat feet," Peter said. "I went to a foot doctor who made some custom-made arch supports for me. They were made out of some type of hard plastic and were just too difficult to walk on. I finally quit using them. They really didn't help—and they were extremely expensive."

"It sounds like you had a bad experience. How did the podiatrist measure you for them?"

"He made a plaster cast of the bottom of my foot."

"Were you lying down, sitting, or standing when he did it?"

"I was sitting down while he molded the plaster around my foot and then let it dry. I picked up the inserts a couple of days later. The whole thing was a complete waste of money."

I imagined it might be difficult to persuade Peter to buy a new pair of orthotics. "There's no doubt you need arch supports," I said. "I'll do things much differently, however. First, when I take a mold of your feet, you'll be standing. It's important to cast your feet while they're bearing weight—that's when you need the support, not when you're sitting or lying down. Second, I'll send the molds to Foot Levelers, a company in Roanoke, Virginia, that's been manufacturing this type of support for more than fifty years. As far back as the 1950s, when I practiced in Minnesota, I ordered from them. Many years ago, I attended a seminar led by Dr. Monte Greenwald, the company founder and a chiropractor, who stressed that proper foot balance is essential for a healthy spine. He developed *Spinal Pelvic Stabilizers*—soft, comfortable leather and rubber orthotics."

Peter's silence emboldened me to continue. "I *do* agree, orthotics can be expensive, but I assure you it's money well spent. I have only your best interests in mind when I urge you to make this investment for your health." I paused. "So . . . what would you like to do?"

"Hmm." Frowning, Peter folded his arms across his chest and stared at the floor. He stewed that way for several moments. Just as I began to wonder if he was going to repeat his performance from the first visit, he dropped his arms and looked up, nodding. "Okay . . . let's do the casting."

Without hesitating, I took molds of his feet, completed the necessary paperwork, and mailed everything to Foot Levelers. When the orthotics arrived the following week, Peter and I checked their fit in his shoes. "These are really comfortable," he said, sounding surprised. "I can actually feel like I'm standing taller and straighter. I'm impressed. They may not stop my shoulder pain, but I do know they make my feet feel much better."

"I'm confident they'll make a difference. It's clear the fallen arches created several changes throughout your body. Your flat feet forced your knees to rotate inward, leading to an abnormal twisting of the femur—the long thigh bone—which changed the way your pelvis had to adapt. The shift in your pelvis weakened the psoas muscles. The pelvis is the foundation of the spine, and when your pelvis shifted, the spine also had to shift to accommodate. An abnormal positioning of the vertebra—a subluxation—caused the stabbing pain in the back of your shoulder. My adjustments would correct the subluxation, and then running with fallen arches undid the correction. And that brings us back to where we began—to your feet."

"So now let's test my muscles with the shoe supports," Peter said, lying down on the adjusting table. Just as I would have predicted, the psoas muscles tested very strong.

"These insoles were a bit expensive, but they sure were worth it. They feel fantastic and make my muscles stronger. They'll probably improve my workouts too."

I adjusted Peter's spine and corrected every subluxation. "Wear the orthotics continuously for the next week," I said. "They'll fit in all your shoes. Go running on Sunday as usual. Make an appointment for next Monday, and we'll check everything then."

When I saw him after the weekend, Peter greeted me warmly. "I'm doing really well," he said, shaking my hand. "The supports don't hurt my feet, and the intense pain in my shoulder blade is completely gone. I'd like to thank you for two things: First, thanks for getting rid of that nagging pain. And second—the most important thing—thanks for pointing out I needed to readjust my priorities and spend money on my health, and not just on looking good. You know, I'm wearing the orthotics all the time. In fact, I want to order another pair so I'll never have to be without them."

Amazingly enough, Peter ultimately purchased orthotics for his boots, his sneakers, and several other pairs of shoes. Since that time,

Foot Levelers has designed dress shoes, sport shoes, and sandals with custom-made orthotics built right in.

The body is a wonderfully designed structure with an innate ability to adapt and compensate for the discrepancies that develop throughout its lifetime. Pain is merely a message that something is wrong. Its source may be at the site of the discomfort, or it may stem from a different, remote place. No matter where it is located, pain should not be ignored. Please see your chiropractor.

12

The Bed-Wetting Secret
Embarrassing Problem Solved

> With God, all things are possible.
> *Matthew 19:26*

In the small town of Olivia, near the county hospital where my first son was born, Timothy O'Riley owned and operated a bakery. His shop was a favorite of mine, and whenever I was in the area, I'd treat myself to one of his doughnuts or apple turnovers. One day Tim surprised me by appearing in my office. He told me he'd been suffering from severe lower back pain for some time. Evidently, his daily chore of lifting heavy bags of flour had seriously overtaxed his body.

Upon examining Tim's spine, I discovered he had a restricted range of motion (ROM). When I asked him to bend *laterally* (to the right and then to the left), I saw that his spine was inflexible in the lower three vertebrae—L3, L4, and L5. The point at which he started to bend was four to five inches higher than normal. His range of motion totaled only sixty degrees from right to left, considerably less than the healthy range of eighty degrees.

After the exam, I led Tim to the x-ray room. X-raying the lower back usually entails taking two views: *lateral* (from the side) and *anteroposterior*, or A/P (directed from the front to the back). To evaluate his limited motion, I included two additional pictures: one in which he was bending to the right and the other, to the left.

In the early years of my practice, before the invention of the automatic processor, I hand-developed x-rays. For each film, I followed five steps: (1) clip the film into a hanger and dip it in the developer for five minutes, (2) wash it in the central tank of water to stop the developing process, (3) dip it in the fixer for five minutes to stabilize the emulsion on the film, (4) wash the picture again, and (5) hang it up to dry. Generally, the patient had to wait more than an hour while I developed all the films and studied them on the view box.

When reviewing x-rays, medical doctors check for fractures, complete dislocations, tumors, changes in bone density (*osteoporosis*), and other gross findings. Chiropractors routinely look for these conditions *and* include others often ignored by physicians, for instance, factors related to bending motion. Lateral bending requires a *coupled motion:* as the spine bends to one side, the vertebrae actually rotate toward the opposite one. Tim's x-rays clearly showed that his lower back was locked up and did not rotate normally when he bent from side to side.

I explained my findings to Tim and outlined a program to correct his condition: We would begin each appointment with two physical therapy modalities—*intersegmental traction* to increase vertebral flexibility and stability, and *diathermy* (deep heat) to relax the musculature—and then we'd move on to spinal adjustments. Within just a few visits, both Tim's pain and range of motion had improved, enabling him to resume his chores. After he fully recovered, I discharged him and did not see him professionally for several years. (Of course, whenever I was in Olivia, I'd stop at his bakery and buy something to satisfy my sweet tooth.)

Close to a decade later, Tim returned to my office. I assumed he had reinjured his back. When I greeted him, he stared down at his feet and seemed embarrassed. "Uh. . . Dr. Rude . . . uh . . . can chiropractic do anything for bed-wetting?" he finally blurted out.

Startled, I asked, "When did you start having a problem?"

"Oh no, it's not me—it's my son, Gary. He graduated from Olivia High School in June and enrolled in the pre–seminary course at St. John's for the fall. He's a good student—always on the honor roll—and he held a class office during his junior and senior years. Gary's a great kid, was popular all through high school. But all this time, he's been living with a secret—he wets the bed. It's been going on since he was a small boy. And my wife is such a saint. Every morning, she strips off the sheets and washes them, and then remakes the bed with fresh linens."

He paused and took a deep breath. "You know, Gary has always dreamed about becoming a Catholic priest, but this morning he told us he's not going to college. He is so terrified about living in a dorm and sharing a room with someone who'll find out he wets the bed."

Tim's eyes filled with tears. "That's one helluva burden to carry around. We kept praying things would get better, that he would outgrow it. . . . What a terrible cross for a young guy to bear." His sadness hung heavily in the air, and my heart went out to him.

My first goal was to ease his mind. I dug out a copy of a "Dear Abby" column titled "Fifteen-Year-Old Bed Wetter Cured by Visit to Chiropractor" and handed it to Tim. When he finished reading, he looked up, visibly relieved.

"Yes, chiropractic *can* successfully treat bed-wetting, Tim," I said. "Let me explain: The brain is in charge of supplying the energy that flows through the spinal cord. Branching off the spinal cord are sets of nerves that pass between the twenty-four vertebrae of the spinal column and out into the body. Each nerve carries vital energy and information to the cells of its designated gland, organ, or tissue. And leaving every cell are nerves that transport information back to the spinal cord and up to the brain. As a result, all the cells in the body have a two-way communication with the brain, except free-floating blood cells. When a misaligned spine interferes with the normal transmission of nerve impulses, something in the body malfunctions. In your son's case, I suspect the typical bladder's message of 'Gary, wake up, I'm full and it's time to go to the bathroom,' is not traveling to the brain."

"I'm not sure I follow you exactly. . . ."

"Hmm, let's see. I'll give you an example: If you'd like to wiggle your big toe up and down, your brain sends an order to the muscles that do the wiggling. The thought creates a message that travels all the way down the spinal cord to the fifth lumbar nerve—that's the nerve branching off between the last vertebra and the pelvis. The message then passes down the leg nerve to the muscles controlling the toe's movement. Other nerves follow a similar trip in reverse—they begin in the skin, ligaments, and muscles of the big toe, travel up the leg, enter the spine at the fifth lumbar vertebra, and go up to the brain. This intercommunication is responsible for the sensation you feel and interpret as your toe's wiggling. It's also the reason you feel pain when you smash or stub your toe. I believe Gary's difficulty lies in the return path. There is a short circuit somewhere, and crucial information is not reaching the brain."

He nodded. "Okay, I'm starting to understand."

"And there's something really simple I can do to check this," I continued. "On both his right and left sides, one of the nerves connecting to the bladder also connects to the big toe. I predict Gary's big toe muscles will be weak. That's because of an interesting fact: When a spinal misalignment shows up as a nonfunctioning organ—in this case, your son's bladder—the strength of the muscles sharing the same nerve supply—the big toe muscles—is reduced. If one branch of the nerve is affected, chances are other areas fed by the same supply will also be affected. Therefore, once I adjust the appropriate vertebra, not only will Gary's toe be stronger, but, more importantly, his bed-wetting will disappear as well."

Tim's face brightened. "It sure sounds like you can help him. How soon can I bring him in?" We scheduled an appointment for his son to come in the next day.

When I met Gary, I saw a handsome six-footer with blond hair and blue eyes. As we talked about his delicate problem, he blushed and fidgeted in his seat. He admitted he'd never been able to accept a sleepover invitation from a friend, something that had tormented him for years. Eager to alleviate his suffering, I briefly described the nervous system and the solution chiropractic could offer.

"Do you really think this'll work?" he asked.

"Yes, there's a very high probability. We'll know more after the exam."

He sprang out of his chair. "Well, let's get started right away—what do we do first?"

The examination confirmed my suspicions. Gary's *flexor hallicus longus* (the large toe muscles) showed weakness on both sides. After the physical exam and x-rays, I adjusted his spine at the L5 and T12 vertebrae (the L5 nerve tells the base of the bladder to contract and squeeze out the urine; the T12 nerve communicates the need to urinate with the brain). I told him to make another appointment for the next day. Gary was scheduled to leave for St. John's the following week, so we had to work quickly—I had only seven days to correct his spine. I adjusted him daily except Sunday until he left for college. Two days before his departure, he rushed into my office. "I didn't wet the bed last night!" he shouted, beaming.

I adjusted his spine twice those final two days and then one last time when Gary stopped into the office on his way to St. John's. He had been dry for three consecutive nights and felt confident that his problem was finally over. He saw me for a checkup on the first weekend he returned home, and happily reported he hadn't had a single embarrassing accident.

I'll always remember the last morning before he went off to school. He shook my hand and warmly expressed his gratitude for what I had done for him. Just before leaving, he said, "May God bless you, and may God bless everyone who visits you for your healing hands."

We now address Gary as Father O'Riley. Thanks in part to chiropractic, he was able to fulfill his dream and has helped thousands of people through the work of God.

13

Susan's Ideal Complexion
Healing Without a Scar

> The preservation of health is a duty. Few people seem conscious that there is such a thing as physical morality.
> *Edmund Spencer*
> *(1552–1599)*

On a Sunday in August 1981, my wife, Shirley, and I were awakened by an early morning phone call. It took me a few seconds to recognize my receptionist's voice. "I was in an accident last night," she said, "and I won't be able to come to work tomorrow morning. You and Carla will have to do without me for a few days." I could tell she'd been crying.

"How badly were you hurt?" I asked.

"Oh, well . . . I guess I'm okay—no broken bones or anything like that. It's just that . . . the whole left side of my face looks like raw hamburger."

Her news jolted me wide awake. Susan was a beautiful young woman—a perfect smile, radiant skin, big brown eyes, and waist-length hair. If the accident had badly damaged her face, permanently scarring her, she would be shattered.

"Gosh, what happened?"

"I got run over by a truck. . . . I'll probably be in the hospital until Wednesday."

(At that time, the nurses and physicians—not the insurance companies—dictated when a patient was well enough to be discharged. The staff was allowing Susan ample time in the hospital. Today, on the contrary, insurance companies demand a rapid release to minimize costs.)

"Can you have any visitors?"

"Yes—and I'd really like the company."

"Shirley and I will be there as soon as we can. We still have to get dressed and have breakfast. You can tell us the rest of the story when we see you."

"Okay, I'll be expecting you. By the way, would you mind doing me a favor? Could you please stop at the office on the way and pick up a bottle of NutriWest's vitamin E? I want the 400 milligram oil capsules, not the dry tablets."

"Sure thing. We'll help in any way we can."

We found Susan in room 241 at the Boulder Community Hospital. A large bandage covered the left side of her face. When she saw us, she gave us a pained half smile.

"You were run over by a *truck*?" I asked, still shocked.

"Yeah, hard to believe, isn't it? You see, every Saturday night, Howie and I—you've met Howie, my boyfriend?—well, we usually go dancing at the Hilo Club and then he takes me home. Last night, Howie was using the van, the one he drives for Frito Lay when he's making his deliveries. There are two bucket seats in front, and the back is wide open with shelves for stacking the snacks, but they were empty last night." She paused to take a sip of water.

"You know how hot and dry it's been? Well, the van has no air conditioning, so we rolled down both front windows, and Howie opened up the big sliding door on the passenger's side to get more air flowing through. As we were heading down Folsom Avenue, I started brushing my hair. I dropped the brush behind the seat, and I stood up and turned around to pick it up. Just then the van swerved, and I lost my balance—and fell out the door. I landed flat on my stomach with my head pointed to the right. Howie slammed on the brakes and backed up, and the rear wheel went right over me. When he heard the thud, he panicked and drove forward again—and ran over me a *second* time."

It was a blessing Susan had been lying face down. Apparently, the wheel had passed over her left shoulder, across her back, and down off her right hip. Had she been on her back, however, the van's weight would have probably fractured her ribs. Nevertheless, her face had been dragged across the pavement, and little gravel pieces and other debris had become embedded in her left cheek.

"The doctors in the emergency room checked me over really well," she said. "Nothing was broken. My midsection is sore and my ribs hurt some. All in all, I guess I'm pretty lucky. . . . The only problem is the left side of my face." She undid the bandage. The rough cement had scraped the flesh almost to the bone. The nurse had meticulously cleaned and disinfected the area, then applied a thick greasy lotion, similar to the ointment used for severe burns. Almost the size of a large ladling spoon, the mutilated skin did look like a piece of meat—covered with transparent gravy.

"The doctor told me I'll have a scar, but if I keep it covered with this ointment, it shouldn't be too bad. He said I can always cover it up with make-up. I want to try something else, though. I don't think this Vaseline-like stuff will work as well as vitamin E, which I've discovered is very healing for the skin."

She tossed her covers aside and sat on the edge of the bed. "At the office you have a book about vitamin E by Dr. Shute. He writes about a little boy who was riding his bike when a truck hit him. He got pinned underneath and was dragged until the truck stopped. I read that his clothes and most of his skin were scraped off. Dr. Shute treated him with vitamin E, and the boy had only minor scarring. My situation is not as bad as his, so maybe I'll have the same results—or even better."

Susan walked gingerly to the wash basin. After carefully washing her cheek, she punctured a hole in a vitamin E capsule with a large pin from her purse. She squeezed out the oil and applied it to her macerated cheek, needing half a dozen capsules to completely cover the area. When she returned to bed, she seemed pleased. Her self-prescribed medication appeared to have restored a measure of optimism.

For several years, Susan had been my right hand *and* arm at the front desk in my office. She handled nearly everything—the appointments, phone calls, insurance matters, and collections. When I recommended vitamins for treatment, she was the one who dispensed them to the patients. She had started reading my reference books to learn about supplements. I appreciated her industriousness because she could answer most of the patients' questions without interrupting me. And now she felt confident enough to apply that knowledge to her own situation.

Shirley and I stopped by the hospital again the next day and found Susan in good spirits. "The nurse changed the dressing this morning," she said. "She cleaned the area and applied the same greasy lotion. But right after she left, I washed my cheek and spread vitamin E on it again. I told her later I thought it would heal better without a bandage pulling on the scab, and also being open to the air might speed up the healing. The nurse agreed, which surprised me. Now I can put the vitamin E oil on it throughout the day."

When I saw her over the noon hour on Tuesday, she told me the doctor was pleased with her fast recovery and would be sending her home that afternoon. "Still, I don't think I should come to work looking like this," she said.

Susan continued her self-prescribed therapy and returned to work the following Monday. Her left cheek appeared pinker than normal, yet it had healed and no longer had a scab. By the end of the second week, I couldn't tell she had been injured. There was never much of a scar, and even upon close examination, I could see only a very slight hint of the accident.

"Vitamin E is a remarkable supplement," I said. "I'm sure you've found out that it does a lot more than just treat the skin?"

"Yes, it does. You know those mailers from NutriWest in Wyoming? I always study them to find out as much as possible about nutrition. I read that Vitamin E is a powerful antioxidant, and it's fat soluble, so you should take it with other fats to make it absorbable. It slows down aging, prevents cancer and heart problems, and increases oxygen to the body, which helps lower fatigue. It also guards against leg cramps. In his *Vitamin Bible*, Earl Mindell says vitamin E is particularly important for women because it reduces the problems connected with PMS, birth control pills, pregnancy, and menopause. And I learned that the trace mineral selenium increases its effectiveness. I'll sure be taking vitamin E for the rest of my life."

I told her how impressed I was with her taking charge of her health, and by working so hard to learn more, she had become invaluable to my practice.

"Come to think of it, Susan, you deserve a raise. You'll find an extra dollar per hour in your next paycheck."

14

Excruciating Eyeball Pain
Introduction to Cranial Adjustments

Don't say you've tried everything unless you've tried chiropractic.

Rosalita Hernandez
Massage Therapist

As a general rule, I don't see patients on Thursday afternoons. Instead, I usually reserve that time for relaxing and maybe playing a round of golf. I do remember, however, one particular Thursday in the early 1970s when I was more than willing to make an exception.

Shortly after noon, my assistants left for the day and I locked up, ready to head out to the golf course and enjoy the Colorado sunshine. Just as I reached my station wagon, I saw a car with Nebraska plates enter the parking lot. At first I thought the two women were looking for a place to turn around, but when they pulled up next to me, I decided they probably needed directions.

"Are you Dr. Rude?" asked the driver as she rolled down the window. When I nodded, she said, "Oh, good. Hannah Kroeger told us to come see you."

I had heard of Hannah, but I'd never been formally introduced to her. Well known in Boulder, she was a combination herbalist, guru, lay minister, faith healer, witch doctor, and owner of a health food store. Her special tonics, and publications and seminars on herbs helped many people when orthodox medicine failed. Word of Hannah's success had spread nationwide.

EYEBALL PAIN

The woman whipped open her door. "I'm Rosalita Hernandez," she said, thrusting out her hand, "and this is Irene Toste." She turned to her companion, who was slowly making her way around the car. "Are we ever glad we caught you before you drove off. We're from Broken Bow, Nebraska. I do massage and reflexology, and Irene came to me for the horrible pain she has in her left eye."

"We arrived here—"

Rosalita talked right over her friend. "I tried all the reflex and acupressure points I know that are related to the eye, but they didn't relieve the pain. I told Irene we needed to drive to Boulder, Colorado, to see my friend Hannah Kroeger. Hannah does things very differently than any other healer I know. I thought she could come up with a solution."

"We arrived here from Broken Bow last Sunday," Irene managed to finish. "Since it's a long drive—about 350 miles—we stayed at Hannah's place overnight and saw her Monday morning." She was referring to the large cement-block building where Hannah conducted classes and offered special healing sessions. She had equipped the second floor with small sleeping rooms to accommodate out-of-town clients and visitors. "I met with her every day this week," she went on, "but after my appointment this morning, Hannah admitted she wasn't getting anywhere with my problem. Then she recommended I see you and—"

"Hannah spoke very highly of you," Rosalita interrupted again. "She said she hadn't met you, but she'd heard you've done some wonderful things. As long as we've come this far, I thought we should at least *talk* with you." Despite her small size, Rosalita was a powerhouse, unafraid to take charge.

Mrs. Toste put her hand up to her eye. "Oh, please help me get rid of this awful pain," she pleaded.

"I'll sure do my best. Come on in. I need to take your history to learn more about your problem."

Irene explained she'd had eyeball pain for more than four and a half years, beginning shortly after a traumatic car accident. Her husband, the owner of the Broken Bow Chevrolet dealership, had died instantly. She didn't recall hitting her head during the collision, and she was certain she hadn't lost consciousness. Shock and grief had erased some of her memory, although she did know her eye started to hurt within a couple of months of the accident.

"The pain is constant," she said. "It feels like a knitting needle is boring into my eyeball. Sometimes it's worse, sometimes it's better, but it's always there."

"What kinds of treatment have you received?" I asked.

"Well, first, I saw my local physician in Broken Bow, who prescribed Percodan, which did nothing. Next, I saw a doctor in North Platte—that's a larger city near Broken Bow—but he couldn't help me. Then I went to an ophthalmologist who gave me another painkiller—Demerol. And again, no relief. I tried doctors in Kearney and Grand Island, and I even went to the medical college at the University of Nebraska in Lincoln. Each time, they gave me a different drug—Darvon, Naprosyn, Fiorinal—but nothing stopped the pain."

She also visited a neurologist at a large clinic in Omaha. "He said it was obvious that drug therapy wasn't the way to treat my problem. The only other thing he could recommend was removing the eye. And I would have agreed to surgery if he had guaranteed an end to my pain, but he couldn't do that. I didn't want to be disfigured if it wasn't going to work. . . . I've spent over *thirty thousand dollars* trying to get some relief. I just don't know . . . how much longer I can . . ." Her breath caught and she couldn't continue.

I wanted to reassure her somehow. "Irene, once I do a complete examination and take some x-rays, I may be able to make some suggestions."

Throughout our conversation, I'd been carefully studying her facial contours. I noticed a great disparity between the two sides of her face, leading me to believe she had distorted *cranial* (skull) bones and probably subluxations in her upper neck, all of which could contribute to the type of pain she described.

During the exam, I found considerable muscular tension at the base of Irene's skull, especially on the left side. And when I palpated an area *under* the base of her skull, the extreme tenderness made her jerk away from my hands. This evidence further supported her having *cervical* (neck) misalignments.

Then, with a rubber glove on my hand, I inserted a finger into her mouth and checked the *infratemporal fossa* (the small pocket on both sides of the mouth between the outside of the upper back teeth

EYEBALL PAIN

and the inside of the cheek). This area was very tender as well. "When you barely touch that spot, it makes the pain worse," she said, confirming my suspicions she also had cranial distress.

To best communicate my findings with her, I instructed Irene to stand in front of the mirror. "I want you to imagine a dot in the center of your forehead right at the hairline," I said. "Now, visualize another dot in the middle between your eyebrows. Then place a third dot on your upper lip, in the center under the septum of your two nostrils, and imagine the last dot in the middle of your chin, again right in the center. Look at all four dots—they should make a straight line. But you actually have a curve, with the inside on the left side. I refer to this as a 'banana head.'"

"Dear God, my face is in an awful mess, isn't it? How could I have missed that?"

"Don't be too hard on yourself. Unless you know what to look for, it's not that easy to spot." I picked up her chart. "Let's go down the hall and continue the exam with a series of x-rays." The skull pictures didn't reveal anything new beyond the facial distortion I'd already observed. The neck films were far more helpful, providing visual proof that the upper two cervical vertebrae, C1 and C2, were misaligned—the source of the tenderness at the base of Irene's skull.

Pointing at the neck x-rays, I explained, "Nerves emit from the spinal cord at the level of these vertebrae and supply the short muscles from the neck to the skull. They're the ones that help balance your head on top of your neck. The displaced vertebrae are disrupting the nerve flow to those muscles, making them contract more on the left side than the right. This contraction is distorting the shape of your skull, contributing to the banana-head appearance."

"So you're saying it's actually my tight neck muscles that are causing my eye pain?" she asked, slightly puzzled.

"Yes, but that's not the whole story. The tenderness in your mouth has convinced me you also have skull bones out of alignment. The eight bones that make up the skull—the *frontal*, two *parietals*, two *temporals*, the *occiput*, the *ethmoid*, and the *sphenoid*—completely encase the brain. Attached to these bones are a number of jaw and facial bones. The eyeball socket is comprised of mostly facial bones, but the frontal and temporal bones on each side of the skull are also involved. One end of the muscles that move the eyeball is attached to the bony socket structure and the other end is attached to the eye itself. The skull distortion is stressing the bones and muscles around your left eye, leading to the extreme pain."

Irene reached out and touched my arm. "Since you seem to know what's wrong, is it possible you can fix it?" Her eyes begged for some good news.

"I'm confident I can provide some relief—at the very least."

In order to give her the best possible adjustments, I needed to start with the cervical subluxations. As Irene lay on her back on the adjusting table, I repalpated the problem vertebrae in her neck and carefully positioned my fingers on the area that needed adjusting. Then I rotated Irene's head to the side and delivered a short, sharp thrust. I felt the movement between the two spinal segments, and I knew she not only felt it but also heard a loud popping.

She jerked away from my fingers. "Wow! That was really strange—but it didn't hurt."

"The noise is normal," I said, reaching for her head and cradling it in my hands. "The vertebrae make that kind of sound when they move back into their proper positions." When I felt the taut muscles at the base of her skull softening, I started gently massaging her neck to promote further relaxation. I wanted her to be as totally relaxed as possible before adjusting her skull.

Then again with a rubber glove on my hand, I reached inside her mouth and placed my index finger on the infratemporal fossa. Irene told me it didn't hurt as much this time. To relieve any remaining discomfort, I adjusted the flat facial bone called the *vomer* (the bone above the infratemporal fossa) by applying pressure opposite to the direction that caused the intense pain during the exam. Similarly, I adjusted the *sphenoid* cranial bone in the roof of Irene's mouth by placing my finger on it and pulling upward.

Irene looked up at me from the adjusting table. "The pain is completely gone," she said, stunned.

Because Irene had expressed apprehension about her first chiropractic experience, Rosalita had stayed in the room the entire time. Upon hearing Irene's announcement, she jumped up and clapped. "Goody, goody, goody!" she shouted.

They agreed to return on Friday so I could make sure everything had stayed aligned. They left the office and I locked up for the second time that day. I hadn't gone golfing, but I did feel enormously satisfied for accomplishing something that had challenged the best of the medical profession.

When I saw my two ladies the next day, Irene told me the eye pain had not returned. I put on a rubber glove and reexamined her infratemporal fossa. "It's tender, but not very much," she said. "I can't believe the change could be so huge so quickly. I've been suffering with it for such a long time."

I palpated her neck and found some residual muscle tightness. "Irene, I've fixed the symptom that brought you to see me: the pain in the eyeball. In chiropractic, however, we don't settle for just relieving the symptoms, we want to remove the cause. Do you feel the tightness in your neck muscles? If left unattended, it could become much worse and pull the same bones out of place, bringing back your pain. I'll adjust your neck again to try for a more perfect correction."

Considering it was at the end of the work week, I assumed Irene and Rosalita would be heading back to Nebraska the following morning. Taking a lead from her assertive friend, Irene spoke up. "If there is still something wrong that needs to be worked on, I think we should stay over until tomorrow for one more adjustment. I don't want to make the mistake of fixing it only partway. Then I'd have to come all the way back again. Do you happen to have office hours on Saturday?"

"Usually not, but if you're willing to stay another day, I'm certainly willing to come to the office in the morning and give you one last checkup. I'll meet you here at nine o'clock. That way, you can still get on the road early enough to make it back to Nebraska by midafternoon."

They were waiting in the parking lot when I drove up at nine. The reexamination revealed minor cervical muscle tension, but everything else was normal. I adjusted her neck and urged her to see the chiropractor in her hometown.

On her way out, Irene stopped at the front desk, brought out her checkbook, and asked, "How much do I owe you?"

I looked her right in the eye and answered with a straight face, "You owe me thirty thousand and *one* dollars."

Her eyes nearly popped out of her head. "*What* did you say?"

"Well, I figure that success should be worth more than failure, and you said you'd already spent thirty thousand dollars."

She started to speak then stopped and smiled when she realized I was just kidding. "You're absolutely right. I *do* owe you more than all the medical doctors combined. They took all the money I had from the sale of the car dealership, and now I'm on Social Security and Medicare."

"In that case, we'll send the bill to Medicare."

She took my hand in both of hers. "Thank you," she said, "and thank God there's such a thing as chiropractic."

Author's Note:

Not all of my colleagues have studied cranial work. I learned how to adjust the cranial bones in a postgraduate class. This valuable technique can successfully treat not only eye problems and headaches but also dizziness, sinus conditions, balance difficulties, *bruxism* (tooth grinding), throat and jaw problems, and ringing in the ears, to name just a few.

15

The Big Fat Guy in the Reception Room
A Case of High Triglycerides

The five most dangerous words in the English language are "maybe it will go away."

Rolla Pennell, D.C.
Clinic Masters Seminar

In looking back over the years and thinking about all the patients I've helped, I'm reminded of a phrase I often use: "Someone up there looks after me." Speaking these words fills me with awe and a sense that a power far greater than I works through me. A remarkable example of this is the following story, a story of seemingly coincidental circumstances that coalesced and probably saved the life of a total stranger.

It begins when I was still practicing in Hector, Minnesota, and a young man named Don Meylor became my patient. He had grown up in the fertile farming area of northern Iowa and married his high school sweetheart. Excited about purchasing a farm, they saved every nickel, but the land in Iowa was just too expensive. Since Minnesota property was more reasonably priced, the young Meylors bought a 160-acre farm a few miles outside of Bird Island, not far from Hector.

Because Don's mother valued chiropractic, she taught her children to consult a D.C. first whenever they were sick. She used to say,

"If the chiropractor can't help you, he will refer you to someone who can."

Thanks to his mother, Don came to see me in 1957 for a minor lower back sprain. Soon I was treating his wife and small children. I especially remember his eight-year-old daughter who belonged to the 4-H Club and had chosen pie baking as her project that year. Throughout the summer, she tagged along with her dad to his appointments and always brought me a freshly baked pie.

While I was adjusting him at one of his visits, Don said, "You know, I've wanted to be a chiropractor ever since I was just a boy going to the doctor in Iowa. What exactly would it take to become one?"

"Well, first, you have to pass a two-year pre–chiropractic course that's very similar to pre-med," I began. "Then you must complete a four-year academic curriculum, which includes classes on the body and its functions, on chiropractic, and on performing adjustments. After finishing all the course work, you have to work a full year in the college clinic and take care of patients—essentially on-the-job training. The two state exams are the final hurdle: the State Basic Science Examination that all medical doctors, chiropractors, and osteopaths must pass, and an individual exam by the board of examiners for your specific field."

"Hmm—a little over seven years. You know, now that the price of Minnesota farm land has gone up so much, I'm thinking I could sell the farm and use the profits to put myself through chiropractic college."

And that's what he did. Don enrolled in the Palmer Chiropractic College in Davenport, Iowa, and the Meylor family no longer came to me as patients.

Don's name did not come up again until 1971, a couple of years after I'd moved my practice to Boulder, Colorado. Early that fall, a salesman from a nutritional supplement supply company dropped by. "I'm Bob Abrahamson from Dartell Laboratories," he said, shaking my hand, "and I also represent Met Path Laboratories." Hearing Met Path's name really got my attention since they performed blood testing for doctors and hospitals, and at that time such labs would not do business with chiropractors. (I figured they had adopted this policy out of fear of losing medically related accounts if word spread they were working with chiropractors.)

"I used to work exclusively for Met Path in Iowa," he told me. "Then the new automated blood-testing equipment became available, and I began going around describing it to all the Met Path customers. One of the doctors, a Dr. Meylor in LeMars, turned out to be a chiropractor, which was a big surprise. I admit I hesitated before going into his office. I didn't know that chiropractors could even evaluate a health problem from a blood report."

"Dr. Meylor? Was it *Don* Meylor?"

Bob nodded.

"Gosh, I used to treat his family when I practiced in Minnesota."

'Really? Well, he sure is a nice guy. It seems that one of his patients was a registered nurse who worked at the hospital in Sioux City, Iowa. She agreed to stop at Dr. Meylor's office, pick up the test tubes of blood, and take them to the hospital for testing. She just told them that they were for Dr. Meylor, and that's how his name got on my list." I smiled, impressed with Don's cleverness for figuring out how to work around the system.

"I thought I better clear it with my boss before allowing a chiropractor to be a Met Path client," Bob continued. "When he told me how much business Dr. Meylor was sending through our company, I argued with him to bend the rules—which he did. So I continued making my monthly rounds, checking to see if he needed any medical supplies.

"One time Dr. Meylor pulled me aside and showed me two blood reports of a patient that had been taken one month apart. The first report showed a really high *triglyceride** level of 380, and the second one showed it had fallen to 198—almost normal. I was astounded. As you know, medicine doesn't have a drug for reducing triglycerides like that. I asked him to explain the difference, and he said he had given the patient a nutritional supplement that contains four all-natural substances: *choline, inositol, methionine,* and *betaine hydrochloride.* Because they're *lipotrophic,*† they can help draw the triglycerides out of the blood. He told me this approach works in every case.

---

*Triglycerides are fat molecules that float in the blood stream. With extremely high levels, the fat can plug an artery (fat *embolism*) and cause a heart attack.
†Substances that help increase the utilization of fat.

"I said to him, 'Man, if the drug companies only knew about this combination, the medics would be using tons of the stuff.'

"But he said it can't be patented because all the ingredients are completely natural. There's nothing stopping competitive drug companies from putting a similar product on the market, but they wouldn't be interested in marketing anything that couldn't be protected by a patent.

"After that day, every time I'd stop by his office, Dr. Meylor would show me other tests comparing results before and after he prescribed nutritional supplements. He had such favorable responses that I decided he was onto something. I started reading books about vitamins, minerals, amino acids, fiber, herbs—anything else natural— by authors like Linus Pauling, Adele Davis, Broda Barnes, Emanual Cheraskin. As I became more knowledgeable, I decided I'd become a distributor for a nutritional supplement company. Since Dartell's distributor in Colorado had just recently passed away, I took over his territory."

Knowing the company had an impeccable reputation, I began using Dartell products at the start of my practice. They produce vitamins from natural plant substances and formulate enzyme products from livestock raised without artificial hormones or synthetics. (I had the opportunity to be at the same table during the 1955 National Chiropractic Association convention banquet with Betty and John Robinson and Bill Marquard. John was vice president of Dartell and Bill, the director of sales. So I had a soft spot in my heart for their company.)

Bob's ability to offer lab services as well as nutritional supplements was his foot in the door to most chiropractic offices. He began calling on all the D.C.'s in Colorado, introducing himself, Met Path Labs, and Dartell.

A few weeks after he'd first stopped by, Bob called to tell me I'd be hearing from one of his other customers, a recently graduated chiropractor. Apparently, the first blood specimen this young man had submitted to the lab was taken from a "big fat guy" who was severely overweight. The chiropractor was reviewing the results while the patient sat in the reception room.

"The D.C. panicked when he saw the numbers," Bob said. "You know triglycerides are supposed to be between 120 and 175, right?

HIGH TRIGLYCERIDES

Well, this patient's was over *2000*! He could've had a heart attack right there in the office. He asked me what to do. I said I could tell him, but since I'm not a licensed doctor, his malpractice insurance wouldn't cover him if he took my advice and things went badly. I told him to call you, that you'd be able to help him."

Bob reminded me of the excellent results Dartell researchers had reported for reducing high triglycerides with their product *Lipotrate*. Just then, a call came in on the other line.

"Dr. Rude? Bob Abrahamson told me to call you." His voice was shaking. "I've got this big fat guy in my reception room whose triglyceride level is over 2000. I'm afraid he might be dead when I go out to see him. What should I do?"

"He's going to be fine," I said, trying to reassure him. "I suggest you start him on Lipotrate immediately and triple the recommended dosage on the label. Then do another blood test in three days. Don't expect the level to drop down to normal that fast, but it should decrease significantly. You will also have to put him on a strict diet: almost no fat, especially fried foods; no pasta—carbohydrates should in the form of fruits and vegetables; fish and lean red meats are okay, and so is chicken, but he has to avoid eating the skin because it's loaded with fat."

"Good, okay. I'll go out and talk to him right away," he said, sounding relieved. "I was really worried. . . ."

"I'm sure you'll be pleased with the results. Let me know what happens."

The next time I saw Bob, he told me the patient's triglycerides had steadily declined over five weeks. The first week had been the most dramatic—the first follow-up lab test showed the level had dropped almost one thousand points. The big fat guy's triglycerides eventually returned to normal, eliminating his risk for a heart attack. And, although I never actually saw the patient, I'm confident he lost weight in the process.

Now, what an amazing series of events: A young farm boy from Iowa moves to Minnesota, asks his chiropractor about training to be a chiropractor, and then becomes one. A lab representative becomes involved with natural healing after meeting the young chiropractor. The paths of the two chiropractors from two different states are crossed by that lab rep, and another chiropractor has a patient with high triglycerides whose life was more than likely saved through my intervention. Yes, "Somebody up there looks after me," and, in doing so, He makes it possible for me to help others.

Author's Note:

When Bob Abrahamson commented that medics would be using tons of the same formula Don Meylor used for lowering triglycerides if the drug companies only knew, he didn't know he was being prophetic. The pharmaceutical industry has since developed drugs that do just that, the most common of which is *Lipotor*, a highly advertised product. Almost four pages in the *Physician's Desk Reference* (PDR) are devoted to explaining the drug's details. As with all drugs in the PDR, the known adverse reactions are listed, even if they occur infrequently. More than 2 percent of those taking Lipotor experience chest pain, nausea, bronchitis, *rhinitis* (runny nose), insomnia, dizziness, arthritis, urinary tract infection, and *edema* (water retention). And fewer than 2 percent have reported an additional 121 health problems ranging from dry eyes, leg cramps, and nose bleeds to facial paralysis, irregular heart beat, decreased libido, and high blood pressure. All prescription drugs have side effects, some of which can be serious. The nutritional supplement companies offer approaches that produce the same reaction—lowering the triglycerides—*and* do so without the risk of side effects.

16

Eva's Congestive Heart Failure
Miracles Do *Happen*

> Chiropractic has a philosophy that the body can heal itself if the obstructions to normal nerve flow are removed. Medicine's philosophy seems to be that people are born with too many organs and too few synthetic chemicals.
>
> *Jeffrey Prystupa, D.C.*

Early one morning in the spring of 1970, not long after I had relocated to Boulder, my receptionist stopped me as I was coming out of an exam room.

"There's a woman waiting to see you," she whispered. "She says she has some questions. Her name's Eva Glooster—and she does not look well at all."

When I met Eva, I had to agree. Short and elderly, she had ankles and lower legs swollen to the size of her thighs, the flesh drooping down over the sides of her shoes. Her legs looked like a couple of old-fashioned stove pipes.

"I was wondering if chiropractic could help me?" she asked. "I live in the mobile home park down the street, and when I saw your office, I decided to come in and talk with you."

She told me she had always gone to the medical center. "I've been seeing a cardiologist, Dr. Quigley, for my congestive heart failure. But just the other day he said he couldn't help me anymore—there was nothing else he could do."

That explained the severe swelling. This life-altering condition occurs when the heart muscle loses efficiency and is no longer strong enough to maintain adequate circulation. As the heart's pumping action declines, blood flow to the muscles, tissues, and organs is reduced, seriously compromising the entire body. The situation deteriorates as the heart slowly becomes more ineffective, unable to keep up with ordinary demands.

The problem can reside in the left side, the right side, or in both sides of the heart. When the left side of the heart fails, blood accumulates in the lungs, causing congestion and *dyspnea* (breathing difficulty). When the right side fails, blood backs up into the legs and the liver, leading to problems such as *edema* (swelling), particularly in the legs and ankles; *cyanosis* (bluish skin); liver and spleen enlargement; increased pressure in the veins—visible from prominent veins in the neck and/or backs of the hands; and sometimes jaundice.

The kidneys are also affected. As the heart pumps blood through the kidneys, they must filter and remove waste products, toxic chemicals, and water from the blood. A weakened heart hinders the kidneys from adequately performing their tasks, and excess fluid builds, worsening the edema. At first, a mild swelling develops primarily around the ankles, and then as the body retains more water, the abdomen swells. Eventually all body tissues may swell, including the heart and its surrounding tissue.

"Do you have any difficulty breathing?" I asked.

"I do. I raised the foot of my bed with boards to reduce the swelling in my ankles while I sleep, but that makes it even harder to breathe."

"What medications has Dr. Quigley put you on?"

"He's given me a lot of different ones over the years. I've been taking *Lasix* for a long time."

This drug is a *diuretic*, or water pill. It affects the kidneys, changing the porosity of the *glomerulus* (the filter mechanism), which allows more water and fluids to filter through the kidneys and out of the body. As a result, the swelling decreases, relieving the pressure on the heart. Conventional medicine offers no cure for congestive heart failure, relying on drugs and lifestyle changes (diet and exercise) to improve heart function and relieve symptoms. If the medications fail, or if the cause of the condition remains unknown or unaddressed, the heart will continue to become even less effective.

The diuretic enabled Eva to lead a relatively normal life, but only temporarily solved her problem. As her heart grew weaker, the edema returned, and her physician increased the dosage of her medication. Again, the swelling subsided, but only for a short time. Her condition continued to decline, and the doctor continued to respond by raising the dosage. Ultimately, when that failed to relieve her symptoms, he prescribed a new, stronger drug. And then he increased the dosage of *that* drug.

"Last week the cardiologist told me he couldn't raise the dosage any more or prescribe anything stronger. He said, 'You'll just have to learn to live with it. It'll gradually get even worse. I'm sorry to say it's simply a matter of time.' He wrote down in my records that all his efforts had failed." Eva's voice trembled.

"I live alone—my husband died ten years ago—and I don't want to burden my children or their families. My married daughter and only grandchild live just a few miles away in Longmont. I don't want them worrying about me. I thought I'd buy an emergency life support alarm in case I can't make it to the phone to call for help." She hung her head, her eyes brimming with tears. "Do you think there's *any* chance you can help me?"

I really didn't know—I'd never treated congestive heart failure before. And I hadn't learned any protocol in chiropractic college that dealt with this disease.

"I'll be honest with you," I said. "I'm not sure. I think chiropractic *should* help. You see, every part of the body is controlled by nerve impulses originating in the brain. They travel down the spinal cord and branch out to reach the various tissues, muscles, and organs. I suspect there's an obstruction to the normal nerve energy flow to your heart—that's why it's slowly becoming weaker. The nerves flowing to the heart emit from the spinal cord at the thoracic spine, just below where the base of the neck attaches to the rib cage. I'm talking about this area right here." I reached across and put my hand on her spine at the level of T1 and T2.

"Judging from your unhealthy posture," I continued, "your movement is limited in this area. After years of carrying your head forward, out in front, you've developed a 'widow's hump.' Chiropractic adjustments should free up this area and restore healthy nerve flow to your heart. I'd like the chance to try."

Eva sat quietly for several minutes, staring down at her lap. "I understand," she said, looking up. "You can't make any promises, right?" I nodded and she said, "So now I have to decide if I should spend money on mere speculation." Again, a long silence. "Well, it's only money," she said finally. "My life sure isn't worth living the way it is now, and I know my time is limited. Let's get on with it—how do we start?"

"Let's start with a spinal exam." I palpated T1 and T2 and found virtually *no* movement between one vertebra and the next. Everyone loses flexibility over time, yet there should always be *some* movement, regardless of age. A chiropractic adjustment would create a small amount of motion between them, but it would be minimal. Because her vertebrae were so locked up, she needed a large number of adjustments over an extended period to regain a healthy spine.

Suddenly, I was horrified to think she might die before I could get ahead of her disease. Like a fighter pilot whose damaged plane is plummeting to the ground in a steep dive, would I be able to pull Eva out of danger fast enough? I realized adjustments alone would not be sufficient—the severity of her condition demanded additional therapy.

I remembered a class in my first semester in chiropractic college. The instructor had directed us to pair off—one was to be the patient and the other, the doctor. The patient sat on the exam table while the doctor took his pulse. Using a reflex hammer, the doctor *percussed* (tapped) rapidly over the *spinous process* (the bump that protrudes out from under the skin) of T1 and T2 for about thirty seconds. This stimulation of the spinal nerves to the heart made the pulse rate increase dramatically. Normal pulse rate is between sixty-eight and seventy-two beats per minute, and following the percussion, it rose to more than a hundred. In the same way, I knew I had to increase the stimulus to the nerves that traveled to Eva's heart.

I had an idea: I could duplicate the percussion effect through *electromuscle stimulation* (EMS) by using my *galvanic electrotherapy unit*, an instrument generating a low-voltage direct current that promotes healing when introduced into the body. Applying electrical current to a muscle will make it contract. If the current is set to turn on and off again and again in rapid succession, the muscle will respond by contracting in rapid succession. I explained to Eva that I would place the electrodes of my electrotherapy unit over the muscles on both sides of T1 and T2. Next, I'd set the unit to contract every other second for a total of one minute on one side and shift to do the same on the other, alternating for ten minutes. The contracting muscles would jerk the vertebrae back and forth, stimulating the nerves to her heart. Then I'd follow with a manual adjustment to loosen the fixed vertebrae. I told her daily treatments were imperative for at least two to three weeks, maybe even longer.

"That's okay," she said. "I'll just walk over here first thing in the morning before the swelling gets too bad."

We started her therapy that day. The next morning, and every morning thereafter, Eva was waiting for me when I arrived at the office. Near the end of the second week she told me, "I think it might be helping. It seems to be a little easier to get my shoes on in the morning."

By the end of the third week, I could see small bulges on the outside of each ankle. "Look, your ankle bones are starting to show," I said, wanting to cheer her on. "The swelling is going down. We are definitely making headway."

"I know, and when I'm in bed it's easier to breathe."

"You're losing some of the congestion in your lungs and around your heart, helping your heart work more efficiently." Initially, her blood pressure and pulse had been dangerously high, and I diligently monitored them during each session. I'd noticed they were slowly coming down—another sign that her heart was improving.

After six weeks of treatment, her ankles had returned to normal, so I reduced her appointments to every other day. Eva steadily improved. Gradually we lengthened the interval between visits to one week, then two.

Before long, I pronounced Eva completely recovered. She was adamant about continuing, however. "I'm still going to come twice a month for the rest of my life," she said. "I don't ever want to have heart problems again."

And she was true to her word. During the summer months, she would bring her granddaughter along—to my delight. Young Gloria often insisted they bring me a plate of homemade oatmeal cookies.

Nearly three years later at her regular monthly appointment, Eva said, "I've been doing really well with chiropractic. I don't think I'll need extra care, but in case of an emergency, could you put me in the hospital? My old doctor at the medical center retired and moved to Arizona."

"Eva, I'm really sorry to say chiropractors don't have hospital privileges."

"But what should I do if I have an emergency?"

"You know, I recently saw a cardiologist at the medical center. I needed to have a complete physical—with a treadmill and all the rest—for an insurance policy. I'll talk to him and see if he'd accept you as a patient."

I contacted the physician and he agreed to see Eva. After her meeting with him, she hurried over to my office to tell me what had happened.

"The doctor asked me if I was still taking my heart medication. I told him I stopped when the swelling disappeared. He wanted to know what I'd been doing, and when I said I was seeing a chiropractor, he said, 'Well, you keep right on going to him because he's doing something for you that medicine can't.'" She smiled broadly, excited about delivering an endorsement for chiropractic.

In the spring of the following year, Eva let me know she was thinking of leaving Boulder. "Are there chiropractors in Longmont who do the same kind of treatment you do?" she asked. "There's a brand new retirement facility there, and I was thinking about moving closer to my daughter and her family."

I assured her that I'd help. I made arrangements for her to see a colleague, and she made the move. This happened in 1976 when Eva was seventy-four years old. I never expected to see her again.

I was mistaken.

On Mother's Day in 1997, I had planned to treat my wife, Shirley, to dinner at her favorite restaurant, the Red Lobster. Our two children were living in California and it would be just the two of us, so Shirley invited her friend Louise to come along. This spry ninety-three-year-old woman lived at a nursing home and needed some assistance, but generally she managed well on her own.

Early that evening when we arrived to pick up Louise, she wasn't finished getting dressed, and Shirley went into her room to help. I waited outside in the lobby and passed the time by reading all the signs on the bulletin board. I noticed a list of residents and started reading down the names. I spotted an *Eva Glooster* and did a quick double take—was that *the* Eva Glooster I had treated so long ago?

I said to the head nurse, "I think I might know Eva in room 416—she may have been a patient of mine. Would it possible for me to see her?"

"Sure, I'll take you to her," she said. "But she probably won't remember you—she has Alzheimer's disease. Since it's dinner time now, she'll be in the dining room. We have to lock the door to that area to keep the patients from wandering off."

As the nurse led me down the hall, she told me Eva hadn't been there very long, just a little over three years. When we entered the dining room and walked to Eva's table, I recognized her immediately. Her hair was snow white, her face was very wrinkled, but it *was* Eva. As the nurse had predicted, she didn't remember me, and our conversation was limited because of the Alzheimer's. I stayed only a few minutes.

As we walked out with Louise, I turned to the head nurse and asked, "And how old is Eva now?"

"She turned ninety-five on her birthday in March."

On our way to the car, I couldn't help but think, "Someone up there looks after me." It seemed to be more than a mere coincidence that I was granted yet another opportunity to learn about a patient long after we had lost touch.

During a lecture I attended as a freshman at National College of Chiropractic, Dr. Janse told us, "Depending on how many years you practice, you will perform a number of miracles with your hands." I consider Eva's case to be one of my miracles. I had helped add more than twenty years to her life after the cardiologist had essentially given up, having nothing more to offer. I feel a mixture of pride and awe to have participated in such an extraordinary event—one of the many rewards I've received from practicing chiropractic for more than a half century.

Author's Note:

Now, reflecting back, I wonder why my contrived plan of EMS plus adjustments worked so well. Though I've never read anything about it in chiropractic literature, I do have a theory that might explain its success:

The brain and spinal cord are each covered by tough tissues called the *duramater* and *dural sac*, respectively. Lubricating spinal fluid lies between the brain and the duramater, and between the spinal cord and the dural sac. (To perform a spinal tap for evaluation purposes, a physician inserts a needle into the area between the dural sac and the cord to draw fluid.)

The spinal cord, the spinal fluid, and the dural sac collectively run down the inside of the spinal canal formed by the twenty-four vertebrae, with the dural sac lying right up against the bone. Between every pair of vertebrae is an *intervertebral foramen* (IVF), or opening, into which the tissues of the dural sac protrude in layers called *meninges*. Residing within the meninges are the *nerve roots* (short segments of nerve tissue), which branch outward from the spinal cord and extend into the IVF's outer margin. When the nerves exit the openings to travel throughout the body, they become encased by an insulating sheath and are known as *peripheral nerves*.

The spinal fluid flows from the spinal canal into the meninges and surrounds the nerve roots. Because each intervertebral foramen constantly changes size and shape as the body moves, this fluid cushions the roots from any damage. Unlike peripheral nerves that are maintained by a blood supply provided by the sheath, nerve roots must rely solely on this surrounding spinal fluid for their nutrition. As the body moves and the IVF size and shape change, fresh spinal fluid is actually "squeezed" in and out of the meninges, feeding the roots.

When a subluxation is stuck, causing little to no motion between vertebrae, the normal IVF squeezing action does not occur. As a result, the spinal fluid around the nerve root is no longer replenished, but instead becomes old and stagnant. Robbed of fresh nutrition, the starving nerve root cannot perform adequately. Although it can still conduct the nerve message from the brain to its destination (the heart in Eva's case), the signal is now weaker. Consequently, the tissue at the end of the nerve is impaired, and a disease process begins (Eva's congestive heart failure).

As time progresses, and if the subluxation remains unaddressed, the condition worsens. This chain of events can strike any nerve supply to any organ and may account for many of the slow, undetected illnesses that plague us as we grow older, such as kidney failure, diabetes, and liver disease.

On the other hand, if a fixed subluxation is corrected soon enough and the vertebrae are loose once again, nerve root vitality can be reinstated. Eva's long life demonstrates that a critical condition can be reversed, that good health can be restored—all the more evidence supporting the power of chiropractic adjustments.

17

Betty's Double Vision
It Begins with the Neck

> In chiropractic, the emphasis is on health, wellness, and optimal function, not on the treatment of symptoms of disease.
> *Jack Wolfe, D.C.*
> *President, Northwestern College of Chiropractic*

"Dr. Rude, I have this terrible pain right here. Can you do anything for it?" Betty asked, pointing to the left side of her neck. I noticed she held her head in an odd position, somewhat turned and bent to the left. Her posture looked strange, yet I knew it was probably the most comfortable one she could assume, that it somehow eased her pain.

Medicare adopted an acronym to describe its protocol for determining the need for a chiropractic adjustment: *PART*. The "P" stands for pain, "A" for *antalgia* (bent to one side), "R" for restricted range of motion, and "T" for muscle tone (muscle spasm or weakness). I could see that poor Betty met all four criteria. Even though she wasn't a Medicare patient, her date of birth told me she would qualify for benefits some time soon.

After Betty filled out her medical history, we went into the exam room. Her muscles were in extreme spasm, especially on the left, but even those on the right were tight, contracted to counter the pulling from the other side. As I palpated each vertebra, I found several tender areas in the upper *cervical*, or neck, region. To gather more information for an accurate diagnosis, I led her to the x-ray room and made a Davis series of films.

This series consists of seven views of the head and neck: I begin with two frontal views—one with the mouth closed and the other with it open—in order to clearly observe all seven cervical bones. In a resting position, the *mandible* (jaw bone) lies directly in front of the upper two cervical vertebrae, making it impossible to see the entire neck region with only one film. As a result, the first view (mouth closed) blocks C1 and C2 and shows the lower five vertebrae (C3 through C7). Then for the second view (mouth open), the jaw bone drops down, blocking C3 and C4, and the upper two become visible.

The next three views are taken from the side: First, the patient's head is in the normal upright position; second, the head is bent as far forward as possible; and third, it is bent backward. These views allow the doctor to determine if the vertebrae are fixated (not moving at all) or if they are too loose, slipping backward and forward.

The last two views are taken of the patient's head in an upright position but turned forty-five degrees left of center and then forty-five degrees to the right. Because nerves emit from the spinal cord through openings between adjacent vertebrae at this angle, these films allow the doctor to check the size and shape of each opening, or *intervertebral foramen* (IVF).

I reviewed the films and discussed the results with Betty. "The x-rays confirm that these two cervical vertebrae are out of alignment," I told her, touching the back of her neck below her skull, "which probably caused your muscles to tighten. And that caused *acquired torticollis*, more commonly known as wryneck, or stiff neck. I need to give you an adjustment, but I know it'll be impossible unless we relax your neck first."

We went into the adjusting room, where I directed her to sit on the table. Standing behind her, I instructed Betty to turn her head in the direction her neck was twisted—to the left—just until the pain began to increase. At that point, I raised my right leg and placed my foot next to her on the adjusting table, stabilizing her body with my knee and thigh. I held her head firmly between my hands.

"Now, turn your head hard in the opposite direction—to the right," I said and resisted her efforts for about fifteen seconds. This is a maneuver known as *contralgic contraction*. As the muscles on one side tighten up, the body's built-in neurological mechanism signals the muscles on the other side to relax. By having Betty try to turn her head to the right while I kept it from moving, she actually created tension in the muscles on the right, allowing the severely contracted left muscles in the wryneck to relax.

"Turn your head now and see how it feels," I said.

She slowly moved her head back and forth. "It *is* a little easier to move, but it's by no means gone."

We repeated the procedure a few more times, and each time she gained a little more mobility.

I told her to lie face up on the table. "I'll do my best to adjust you, but since you're so tight, I'm sure I won't be able to do it completely. We can at least begin returning things to normal."

After a fairly successful adjustment, Betty sat up and turned her head from side to side. "That feels much better," she said with a smile. Although still restricted, her range of motion had improved considerably. She made an appointment for the following day.

Upon her return, I rechecked everything and repeated the procedures from the day before. I didn't have to perform as much contralgic contraction, and her neck adjusted much more easily. After a few more visits, Betty was dismissed and resumed her normal routine as homemaker, mother, and part-time accountant.

Several months later, I saw Betty's name in the appointment book. "I have some tension in my neck again," she said, her face lined with worry, "and I'm afraid if I let it go, it'll turn into what I had the last time."

"You made a wise decision."

"Before I came to you, I would get a headache whenever my neck started tightening up. I don't know how to describe the pain exactly, almost like my skull felt tight. It's on the right side, sort of behind my eye. But since you adjusted my neck, I haven't had any problems—not until now."

I palpated her spine and determined that her upper two cervical vertebrae were misaligned again. C1 and C2 subluxations are very common and can cause a host of different complaints, such as headaches, eye problems, tonsillitis, and sinus conditions. I adjusted her neck as I had before, and Betty left the office looking much more relaxed.

I didn't see her again for well over a year. This time she had a different complaint. "I've been getting this funny sensation in my head," she said, "almost like the headaches I usually get, but not quite. I feel a pulling in my right eye, and it seems to be turning outward. I even see double sometimes."

When I studied Betty's face as she lay face up on the adjusting table, I saw a "banana-head" appearance, typical of misaligned *cranial* (skull) bones. (See chapter 14 for an explanation of banana head.)

"Betty, let me explain what's happened. Your problem is still pretty much the same. As I palpate along the base of your *occiput*—that's the bone at the base of your skull—I can feel extremely tense muscles. They're so tight, in fact, that if you weren't contracting your muscles to tilt your head forward, you'd be looking up at the ceiling. This is straining the place where the muscles attach to the occiput. And I can feel that it's much tighter on the right side than on the left."

I rubbed on both sides of the occiput with slightly more pressure to allow her to make a comparison. "Ow!" she cried. "I can definitely feel the difference."

"The muscles that control the eyeball are attached to the eyeball at one end and to the skull bones at the other," I said, massaging her neck, "and these bones are somewhat soft and pliable. The extreme tension in your neck muscles is distorting your skull and therefore disturbing the eyeball muscles. It appears that the muscle turning the eye outward has overpowered the muscle turning it inward. I'm sure the tension you're feeling comes from constantly trying to keep the eye in its normal position."

I told Betty we needed to take another x-ray, but this time it would a bit unusual. "I'll tilt your head way back, place the film at the top of your head, and aim the x-ray at your Adam's apple, pointing upward. This way, I can film the *foramen magnum*—the big hole in the bottom of the skull which the spinal cord passes through—and see the ring of the *atlas*—the bony structure of the top cervical vertebra. I'll also be able to see how the right and left sides balance."

The films revealed two distinct problems: First, Betty's atlas had shifted forward and to the right of the base of the skull; and second, her skull was nonsymmetrical (lopsided), the result of a twisting in the right temporal bone.

Similar to previous visits, I adjusted Betty's first cervical vertebra, C1, which began relaxing her neck muscles. Because these muscles are also attached to the skull bones, as they relaxed, so did the skull bones.

Next, to address her cranial distortion, I had to adjust her right temporal bone internally. With a plastic glove on my hand, I exerted pressure on the back part of the roof of her mouth. Admittedly, working inside the mouth isn't the most pleasant for the patient, but it's a fast procedure and less uncomfortable than dental work. I continued applying pressure until her muscles relaxed and Betty's head returned to normal, losing the banana-head appearance.

I watched her eye swing back to center. "That's utterly amazing," she said. "I can actually feel my eye moving, and I don't see two images anymore. I can't thank you enough. Chiropractic has certainly been a lifesaver."

Betty has been a patient for many years. She comes whenever her neck feels tense or her eye begins to wander. And now, she is old enough for Medicare benefits. Although Medicare recognizes adjustments for only the pelvis, and the cervical, thoracic, and lumbar vertebrae, I do not include an additional charge for the cranial manipulations.

18

A Tale of Two Classes
Chiropractic and Longevity

If I'd known I was going to live this long, I would have taken better care of myself.

George Burns
Comedian

To borrow from Charles Dickens, "It was the best of times. It was the worst of times." The year was 1941, and in early June I graduated from Hector High School. Using money saved from a newspaper route and other odd jobs, I enrolled at the University of Minnesota in the fall and majored in chemical engineering. My whole life stretched out ahead of me, and I eagerly embraced the challenge.

Then, on December 7, Americans were thrown into turmoil when the Japanese bombed Pearl Harbor. Fortunately, college students could apply for deferment if they were studying either medicine or engineering. I applied and was accepted into a navy college training program that allowed me to continue my engineering studies before going into active duty. In 1945 I was commissioned as an ensign, and after serving aboard two ships, I was honorably discharged in 1946.

At that point, I decided to change my course of study and follow in my parents' and grandparents' footsteps. I attended National Chiropractic College in Chicago and eventually transferred to Northwestern College of Chiropractic in Minnesota.

Shortly after graduating in September 1950, I took the Minnesota State Board of Chiropractic Examiners exam to obtain my license to practice. As I sat pondering how to answer the question, Which level of the spine would you adjust to stimulate the adrenal glands in a patient with low blood sugar? I looked up and noticed that all five members on the examination board were senior citizens. Considering Minnesota had passed legislation licensing chiropractors in 1920, these gentlemen must have belonged to the original group of D.C.'s appointed by the governor.

Their actual ages came up in conversation soon after I had passed the exam. I was attending my first Minnesota Chiropractic Association Convention, and during our lunch break, I stopped in at the coffee shop. I spotted my dad, Dr. Harold Rude, sitting with Dr. Barney Lee, one of the board members and a good friend of ours. In fact, Barney and his son, James, visited Hector regularly during pheasant season, and the four of us would trudge through the corn fields searching for the wily birds.

The restaurant was crowded and my dad motioned for me to join them. Soon after, Dr. Curtis, another board member, walked through the door, and Dr. Lee invited him to come sit with us. As we waited for our meals to arrive, Dr. Curtis entertained us with stories of his latest kayaking adventures. Living in Duluth, he frequently ran the rapids in the rivers draining into Lake Superior.

"I paddle out on the water," he told us, "and deliberately flip over the kayak so I'm upside down with my head submerged. And then I practice the maneuver to right myself. It's great fun."

That seemed like quite a feat for a man his age. "How *old* are you?" I asked.

"Seventy-two," he replied, and we started talking about the ages of the other board members: Dr. Konkler, eighty-one; Dr. Kath, late seventies; Dr. Martner, sixty-eight; and Dr. Lee, sixty-five.

No one was tracking life expectancy figures for the years these grand old men were born. At the turn of the twentieth century, a man's life expectancy was 47 years, and in 1923, the year I was born, it had risen to 54.1 years. By the time I graduated from high school, it was 62.9. What could it have possibly been for Dr. Konkler, born in 1869? The board members had clearly outlived all statistics.

I thought of my grandfather, Dr. William Grant Witts, who was also born in 1869. His parents had borrowed his middle name from Ulysses Grant, the Civil War general elected president in 1868. Grandpa practiced chiropractic for forty-four years until his death in 1949 at age eighty. These extraordinary facts helped plant the seed that chiropractic may have something to do with fostering longevity.

Almost twenty years later, after relocating to Colorado, I met Dr. Doerr Belden, a chiropractor from Glenwood Springs, who was eighty-one years old and still practicing. I thought again about the possibility of a link between chiropractic and an extended life.

I gathered more supporting data in 2000 when I attended the fiftieth reunion of my graduating class from Northwestern College of Chiropractic. At the banquet dinner, seating was organized by class, with a placard at each table designating the year of graduation. The class of 1950 numbered more than the ten chairs available, so we spilled over to the class of 1940. Yes, after sixty years, there was one member attending—Dr. Earl Seeliger. When he was asked to say a few words to the crowd, he began, "I am greatly honored to be speaking before you tonight, especially since I am the only member of the class of 1940 who is not in a horizontal position."

Northwestern College of Chiropractic does an excellent job of keeping track of alumni. (Occasionally, I receive a newsletter that describes some improvement they're proposing with an appeal for donations to defray the costs, or an announcement of a memorial fund established in the name of a recently deceased colleague.) At the reunion dinner, each alumnus received a class roster listing current addresses. Of the thirty-one members in my graduating class, only four were followed by the word "deceased." Here again, because so few of my peers had passed on, I wondered about chiropractic's role in extending the lives of those receiving routine adjustments.

Then, at my sixtieth high school reunion in late July 2001, I had the opportunity to study another group of senior citizens. Out of my thirty-two classmates at Hector High, nine were present at the event, nine had other commitments, and fourteen were no longer among the living. So, after sixty years, 44 percent of my graduating class had died.

Comparing my high school and college classes revealed some significant findings. Everyone was approximately the same age, give or take a year, and the group size differed by only one. The college class, however, consisted of men only—important to note because women tend to outlive men. Another major difference had to do with their educational paths: the college graduates were the only ones who had studied the body in its totality. From their chemistry courses at chiropractic college, they had learned about the intricate biochemical reactions occurring in the body that most people take for granted. A Doctor of Chiropractic is trained to look for and analyze minor changes in body structure, function, and chemistry. The laypersons of my high school class of 1941 had not experienced the same education as my fellow D.C.'s.

What do the numbers show? In the year 2000, twenty-seven of the original thirty-one chiropractors, or 87 percent, were still living productive lives. One year later, only eighteen of my thirty-two high school classmates, or 56 percent, were alive. Although this was not a controlled laboratory experiment, I do believe the results are telling.

All the examples I've given are just anecdotal evidence, yet so many octogenarian male chiropractors must say something. Chiropractic emphasizes all things natural and cooperates with the body's innate intelligence and flow of vital energy. It is reasonable to expect that such a philosophy and training would contribute to lengthening a chiropractor's life and the lives of all those who regularly seek chiropractic care. In fact, periodic adjustments, proper nutrition, and other forms of alternative medicine not only increase life expectancy but also greatly improve the *quality* of that life.

19

I'm All Pooped Out
One Solution to Chronic Fatigue

> My medical doctor is my sickness doctor, whereas my chiropractor is my wellness doctor.
>
> *Shirley Spiez*
> *Patient*

A minor automobile accident brought seventy-five-year-old Hildy to my office for the first time in early 2000. "I've never had an accident in my life," she said with a slight European accent, "and I've been driving since I moved to this country in 1948. I suppose this means my insurance will go up. And it wasn't even my fault—*he* ran into me." She paced back and forth, her petite frame slicing through the air.

"How—"

"I've been alone since my husband died," she continued without taking a breath, "and I thought I was handling everything like an expert, paying taxes on the estate and taking care of the house. Now this accident is going to ruin everything."

"So when—"

"I had planned to go on a tour through Europe and see my relatives in Luxembourg, but that dumb guy who didn't obey the stop light has probably forced me to give that up. I am—"

"How did you get a name like Hildy?" I cut in, intent on changing the subject to calm her down.

"Oh." She stopped walking and faced me. "Well, when I was baptized, my name was Hildegarde, but I shortened it to Hildy because I don't like long, drawn-out names. Hildegarde sounds too much like an Old World person, so when I came to America I started out in my new country with my new name." She finally sat down.

I hurried to speak before she started up again. "You probably suffered a whiplash-type injury from your car accident. When and exactly how did it happen?"

"I was driving to the mall where I walk every morning, Monday through Friday. I know exercise is important for maintaining good health, and I am in good shape and want to stay like that. On my way there, I had to stop at a red light and this man ran into the rear end of my car. It made an awful, loud crashing sound—I thought maybe he smashed up my car." She stayed seated, but now her hands began to move as fast as her words. "I knew I had to call the police, so I turned on the emergency blinkers, walked to the flower shop right there on the corner, and called 911. I went back to my car and waited, and then about five minutes later, the officer came. When he saw what had happened, he gave a ticket to the guy who hit me. That stupid young man was driving like a teenager, but I think he was probably in his midtwenties. I hope this won't interfere with my plans for Europe. I have a lot of pain in my neck, and it hurts to turn my head. Do you think you can help me?"

Phew! Could she talk! "Let's see what an examination and x-rays tell us."

After checking her spine and reviewing a complete Davis series of x-rays (see chapter 17 for a description of these x-rays), I was able to reassure Hildy that her whiplash injury was minor, requiring only a few adjustments to correct. "When are you leaving for Europe?" I asked.

"Oh, not until next August. At first, I was going to go in May. You know, the landscape is beautiful in the spring. The tulips are in bloom, and it's just gorgeous. . . ." Her voice trailed off as she turned to the window, lost in thought.

"I think you'll be able to make the tour," I said, bringing her back from her reverie.

She smiled. "Oh, that would make me so happy."

Hildy was an ideal patient, never missing an appointment and religiously following instructions for her at-home rehabilitative care. She asked many questions, always wanting to know what to expect from each adjustment. In a whiplash injury, the ligaments supporting the neck vertebrae are overstretched or possibly torn and, as a result, cannot give proper support to the neck while they're healing. I instructed her to wear a soft foam rubber cervical collar for the first three days, giving the damaged tissue the needed additional support.

The collar can be removed after those three days, but I strongly urged Hildy to wear it while driving to prevent any reinjury if she suddenly had to stop. I also gave her a bottle of Standard Process *Ligaplex I*, a nutritional supplement especially formulated to promote the healing of damaged or injured ligaments.

This supplement opened up a whole new field of study for Hildy. She asked about each component of *Ligaplex I*. I explained, "Manganese, one of the ingredients of *Ligaplex I*, is an essential mineral in the synthesis of cartilaginous tissue and helps maintain the health of ligaments and tendons. The pea vine juice in this supplement is a natural source of many vitamins and minerals needed for the manufacture of *collagen*, a major component of connective tissue. And the ingredient veal bone provides vitamins A, C, E, and B-12, and the mineral phosphorus, all of which are required to make both the yellow elastic fibers and the white collagenous fibers that comprise ligaments."

"What you're telling me," she said, "is all of these vitamins and minerals produce certain effects in the body, and a person can use supplements as a sort of medication for specific conditions?"

"Yes. But like anything you ingest, you can overdo it. Because B and C vitamins are water soluble, your kidneys will eliminate the excess if you take in more than your body needs—but then you have expensive urine. Vitamins A, D, E, and K are oil-based, and your body will store them in the fatty tissues. You can definitely overdose on those. The same holds true for minerals. Certain minerals must be taken in specific ratios to other minerals; if you take too much of one type, you can push your body out of balance."

Hildy fully recovered from the accident and came for maintenance care for several months. She continued to study nutrition, frequenting health food stores and subscribing to every publication relating to her new interest. I marveled at her energy and spunky enthusiasm. For nearly an octogenarian, she was "hell on wheels," still driving her 1981 Audi and bragging it had only forty-three thousand miles on the speedometer.

Her visits to my office eventually tapered off. Almost a year passed before I saw her again, and this time she barely shuffled her 106 pounds into a seat in the reception room. No longer the talkative, vibrant little old lady with a bounce in her step, she looked pale and feeble.

"Hildy, are you feeling okay?" I asked, shocked by her transformation.

"Not really. My health has been going downhill over the last six months." I hardly recognized her frail voice. "I always try to stay active, get plenty of exercise, eat properly, and take my supplements like I should, so I don't know what happened. All of a sudden I started losing energy. Remember how I used to walk in the mall every morning? I can't make it around once before I'm exhausted. I had to take a taxi to come here because I don't think I'm strong enough to drive safely. I'm just all pooped out."

"I'm sure we'll figure out the cause."

She sighed. "You know, Dr. Rude, I eat a good, healthy diet: lots of fruits and vegetables, plenty of whole grains—especially millet—and light on meats and dairy products. I don't eat much different than when I was growing up, the way my mother taught me. And I've been taking vitamins and minerals to make sure I don't get osteoporosis. I take antioxidants to remove any free radicals so I won't get cancer." She seemed to be trying to convince me her fatigue was not her fault.

My ongoing studies of bionutrition repeatedly remind me that good health demands a properly balanced body. When the discovery of the need for antioxidants first hit the media, I was confused by the news. After all, oxygen is vital for life: As soon as we breathe it in, oxygen combines with red blood cells and is distributed throughout the body where it can help produce energy and other body functions. The term *antioxidant* seemed like an oxymoron—why would anyone take something that inhibited the very essence of our vitality?

After investigating further, I learned why we *need* antioxidants—they actually fight the free radicals that can cause cancer. When free radicals were first identified, researchers attributed them to external effects, such as air and water pollution. Today, scientists have confirmed that free radicals are a byproduct of the body's normal metabolism of fats. Usually, the immune system neutralizes free radicals, preventing them from producing cancer; however, over the past couple of decades, Americans have been eating more fats, burdening their bodies with excess free radicals. Since food manufacturers know fats are tasty, they add them to commercially prepared foods to improve flavor and sales. The popularity of fast food restaurants is further evidence of our increased fat consumption.

Just as you can overdose on vitamins and minerals, you can also take too many antioxidants. A research group at Loma Linda University in the late 1990s discovered that excess antioxidants can cause fatigue by interfering with the *Krebs cycle*, a part of the biochemical mechanism that allows each cell to produce its own internal energy.

"Hildy, are you taking a lot of antioxidants?"

"Oh, yes," she said, her face brightening. "I take vitamins C and E, selenium, grape seed extract, CoQ-10, and essential fatty acids. I want all the protection against cancer I can get." At least I'm doing *something* right, her expression said.

"You know, *too many* antioxidants can actually *make* you tired. We all produce free radicals from the fats we eat, but since you're eating a low-fat diet, your body may have fewer of them than the average person's."

"Do you really think that could be possible?" She frowned. "I try to watch my diet carefully, and I take all my supplements on a regular basis. It seems impossible that I've been harming myself all this time. Here I thought I was doing everything I could to stay healthy."

"I know you're very conscientious, but I think we need to consider the possibility. I recommend we check your free-radical levels by running an *Oxidata* test on your urine. I learned about this lab test at a postgraduate seminar in October of 2000, sponsored by Apex Energetics of Santa Ana. They focused primarily on the promising results of free-radical research."

"So how do we run this test?"

"Here's a specimen cup. Don't take vitamins or any other type of supplement for two days. On the morning of the third day, I want you to urinate in this cup—midstream—and bring it to the office along with a completed general health questionnaire. After I run the *Oxidata* test and additional lab tests on both your urine and saliva, we'll have a fairly good report of your biochemical status. We'll determine your level of free radicals, vitamin C, and zinc, to name a few, and also check to see if you're properly absorbing minerals."

Hildy agreed to the tests, and three days later she dropped off her specimen cup and questionnaire. Eager to verify my diagnosis of Hildy's fatigue, I immediately performed the *Oxidata* test. I broke off the top of the premeasured vial and added exactly one cc (cubic centimeter) of urine. After setting it aside for five minutes, I checked its color. If there are no free radicals present, the liquid remains clear and colorless. The greater the number of free radicals, the darker the color—from faint pink to fuchsia to crimson to dark scarlet. Hildy's vial remained as clear as distilled water. Her urine contained no free radicals—just as I had predicted.

When Hildy returned to the office the next day, I had to explain that because the test registered only positive findings (0, +1, +2, +3), we weren't finished. "You see, the fact that your urine showed clear doesn't guarantee things are perfect. It will also be clear for *excess* antioxidants. We'll perform the test again, but this time you need to avoid any form of antioxidant for a week. We're looking for a result that lies between zero and just a faint touch of pink." I gave her another specimen cup and she made an appointment to retest in one week.

After the second round of testing produced the same clear results, I told Hildy, "Just continue without taking any antioxidants for another week, and we'll test again."

The results for the third test were no different. "Let's wait two weeks this time before we test again," I said. Before leaving with yet another specimen cup, she expressed her concern about going four weeks without antioxidants. I urged her not to worry.

Exactly two weeks later, we performed the test for the fourth time, and the liquid still showed no color. Hildy went home with the fifth specimen cup. I didn't immediately throw away the vial, inadvertently leaving it on the lab table while I adjusted another patient.

About five minutes later, I passed by the lab and saw that I hadn't disposed of the vial. When I picked it up, though, I noticed a faint tinge of pink. I quickly called Hildy with the news, adding, "I'm certain the fifth test we run next week will show you're at the optimal level."

When she brought in her next specimen, we both hurried to the lab, anxious for a normal test result. We weren't disappointed this time—a very pale, light pink color appeared in the vial.

"Dr. Rude, it's been five weeks since I took any antioxidants, as you had suggested. I was afraid I'd be low on vitamins C and E, but obviously not, and I feel a lot better. My energy is coming back. It's difficult for me to believe I could have caused myself to be so lethargic and rundown. I'm just thankful I trusted your judgment. I learned the hard way that no one should randomly take supplements without first consulting an expert."

"You're absolutely right. And when you come for your next visit, bring in all the vitamins, minerals, and nutritional supplements you were taking. Based on your lab work, I'll advise you how to proceed from this point forward. You actually may have been missing something that's important."

It wasn't long before she was walking again at the mall and planning another trip to her homeland.

Hildy's story illustrates how critical it is to honor the body, prudently maintaining its biochemistry without overdosing in one area. And it's wise to do so under the watchful eye of an experienced practitioner.

20

Grandpa's Hands
Learning from the Masters

> Go to JAIL for chiropractic.
> *Universal Chiropractic Association*
> *Early 1900s*

As I've mentioned, I have the unusual honor of being a third-generation chiropractor. Both of my maternal grandparents graduated in 1905 from the Keck School of Chiropractic in Nevada, Missouri, and in 1926, when I was three years old, my mother and father graduated in the same class from the Minnesota College of Chiropractic.

While I served in the navy during World War II, Grandma, Dr. Elizabeth Witts, passed away, but Grandpa was still practicing when I returned home. It was his love for chiropractic—and maybe his gentle nudging—that convinced me to follow in his footsteps and carry on the family tradition.

Throughout Grandpa's lengthy career—from 1905 to 1949—he used a vibrator strapped to the back of his hand to give his patients a good rubdown before adjusting their spines. This instrument had an eccentric motor that caused his hand to continuously shake, allowing him to relax the spinal muscles as he rubbed along the back and neck.

Grandpa began having minor fleeting pains in the knuckles of his right hand, so he switched the vibrator to his left. In time, the trauma caused by the continuous vibration affected the joints in both hands. (Today, we know of many conditions that stem from this type of repeated motion. *Carpal tunnel syndrome*, for instance, can develop

101

from overworking the wrist, resulting in pain and numbness in the hand. Workers' compensation claims for on-the-job injuries was a primary reason for the replacement of punched cash registers with infrared scanners. Those doing a considerable amount of keyboard work are also prone to the same problem.)

The pain in Grandpa's hands became too severe, and after forty-four years of soothing patients' muscles and treating their health conditions, he was forced to retire. Eventually, he moved in with my parents. I was attending chiropractic college then, and during one of my semester breaks at home, "Gramps" pulled me aside.

"Kennon, my hands are giving me a lot of trouble—I can't even drive now because I can't grip the steering wheel. I'd like to go to the Mayo Clinic and see if they can do anything for me. If you drive me to Rochester, I'll deed the car over to you—if they can't help me."

I'd heard the stories about the connection between chiropractors and the Mayo Clinic. It seems that the wife of Dr. Charles Mayo, one of the two brothers who had founded the famous medical center in Rochester, Minnesota, had been stricken with some kind of debilitating condition. None of the doctors at the clinic could relieve her problem, and in desperation, Dr. Mayo decided to take his wife to a chiropractor.

To avoid tarnishing the clinic's reputation, they sought help out of state. I've heard two versions of the story at this point. Some say they went to Dr. B.J. Palmer in Davenport, Iowa, the location of the famous Palmer School of Chiropractic. This seems highly unlikely because Davenport is too close to Rochester to protect anonymity. Besides, Dr. Palmer held a reputation for flamboyantly promoting his school and profession, often using his own radio station, WHO, in Davenport as his mouthpiece. (Incidentally, former President Ronald Reagan began his sportscasting career at WHO.)

The more logical version has the Mayos traveling to South Dakota and receiving treatment from either the Tiezens in Marion or the Ortmans in Canistota. Originally from Europe, both were highly reputable families of chiropractors, and both locations were small farming villages about one mile off the main highway, each having a gravel road as the only access to the main street.

The Mayos arrived on a Monday morning and checked into a local hotel. Either Dr. Tiezen or Dr. Ortman adjusted Mrs. Mayo every morning for five days, and on Friday announced her much improved, releasing her to go home. When Dr. Mayo discovered the bill was a mere two dollars a visit—the prevailing fee for adjustments in the days following the depression—he was stunned. "You've got to be crazy," he supposedly said. "You helped my wife when all of medicine couldn't. It's worth a hundred times that much."

The chiropractor responded, "I won't charge you more than any other patient. It's a total of ten dollars."

So Dr. Mayo paid the ten dollars. He also made arrangements to have the town's main street blacktopped as well as the one-mile stretch of gravel road leading in from the highway. Then he took his gratitude one step further: He established a policy at the Mayo Clinic for all chiropractors and their families to receive a free diagnostic examination. (The patient had to pay for any follow-up therapy or surgery.)

Gramps knew about this special perk and desperately wanted to see if the Mayos could fix his hands. I agreed to be his chauffeur, and we drove to Rochester and checked into a motel. At the clinic the next morning, Gramps began the three-day examination, insisting I be allowed to accompany him throughout the entire process. Except for x-rays, I witnessed every procedure, which proved to be an excellent learning experience that I later carried over into my own practice.

Our stay in Rochester gave me a chance to really get to know my grandfather. Even though I'd grown up in Hector, Minnesota, only eighty-five miles from Mankato where my grandparents lived, we seldom spent much time together. Since the highways were not nearly as developed as they are today, driving that distance over graveled roads took over half a day.

After leaving the Mayo Clinic each evening, Gramps and I would stop at a restaurant for a bite to eat and then adjourn to the motel. I know he was proud that I was continuing in the family tradition of natural health care. He seemed excited to pass on some of his firsthand knowledge, entertaining me with stories about his practice.

"Now, I bet you don't know I did some jail time," I remember him saying. "It all started when one of my patients complained about being constipated, and I recommended he drink the juice of a lemon mixed with warm water before going to bed. Pretty harmless suggestion, I thought. But when one of the local M.D.'s got wind of it, he had me arrested and charged with prescribing medicine without a license. The judge actually sentenced me to jail." He shook his head in disbelief. In the early years of chiropractic, medical doctors held a tremendous animosity toward chiropractors—you might describe it as a turf battle.

"While I was serving out my sentence, your grandmother continued seeing her patients. And you remember how she and I shared the same office? Well, my patients started coming in, and she'd tell them I was down the street in jail. She said that since I was allowed to have visitors, they could go see me there. So there I was, adjusting folks on the cot in my cell." We both started laughing.

He said soon there was a steady stream of patients coming every fifteen minutes. "The jailer panicked—he didn't seem to know how to handle all the traffic traipsing through his territory. Well, it wasn't long before the judge stayed my sentence and let me go home."

And then there was the story about one of his patients who suffered an *inguinal hernia* (an abnormal protrusion in the groin occurring most frequently in males). "Loren decided to build a new hog barn," Gramps began. "He'd ordered some asphalt shingles for the roof, and they were delivered to the local lumberyard and stacked outside. It was in the late fall, and before Loren made it into town, we had a light snowfall. The snow melted the next day and ran under the shingles. That night the temperature dropped below freezing, and the bottom of the stack froze to the ground. Loren went to town the following day to pick up his order, and when he bent to lift the last three bales of shingles, they were still frozen to the ground and wouldn't budge. So he jerked harder and suddenly felt a terrible pain in his groin."

Being a faithful chiropractic patient, Loren thought my grandfather could help him out. He managed to get into his pickup and drive over to the office.

"It sure sounded like he had developed a hernia, but I hadn't learned anything in college about treating it. Since I did know how to check for hernias—and I wanted to at least try to do something for him—I told him to drop his overalls, and turn his head to the side and cough. Sure enough, it was a full-blown hernia."

Thinking he should also check his spine, Gramps instructed Loren to lie down on the adjusting table. "I was massaging his back with the vibrator, getting him ready for adjustments, and then I moved down to his thighs. I came to a big knot in the muscle on the inside of his right thigh, about four inches above the knee joint—very strange. His left leg was normal. As I rubbed over the knot, Loren groaned and told me the pain went all the way up to his groin."

Grandpa continued to massage the knot with the vibrator, and it gradually softened. "I worked on that thing for maybe a half hour to forty-five minutes, and I finally got rid of all the tension in his leg. And a funny thing happened—the hernia closed up and disappeared. I don't know why, or what I did, but I was able to help him. Loren continued seeing me for years after that, and the hernia never recurred. You know, Son, I think that's probably one of the most outstanding cases I've ever treated." His eyes lit up with pride.

On our second night in Rochester, Gramps told me, "It must be dull for a young man like you to sit in a motel room with an old codger like me, especially on a Saturday night. Why don't you just take the car and go cruising—maybe you can find a little activity. There must be a lot of young nurses your age out on the town tonight."

I did need a break. I grabbed the keys, and when I headed for the door, he added, "Just remember, if you burn your butt, you're going to have to sit on the blister." I smiled. Those sound words of advice have guided me ever since.

On the third and last day, we sat down with the doctor in charge of my grandfather's case and discussed the results. "Dr. Witts," he said, "all the joints in your hands, fingers, and wrists are arthritic. I'm sorry, but there is nothing we can do. If the pain gets too severe, all I can suggest is taking aspirin." Unfortunately, in 1949 aspirin was the only medication, other than narcotics, available for pain. As we expected, there was no charge for the entire three-day examination.

Disheartened, we returned to Hector. True to his word, Gramps gave me his 1940 Plymouth four-door, which I promptly (and proudly) drove to Northwestern College of Chiropractic in Minneapolis to resume my studies. My grandfather stayed with my folks until he died.

THE MAYO CLINC AND CHIROPRACTORS

Author's Note:

In 1960 I had another experience with the Mayo Clinic. Shirley and I were worried that our four-year-old son, Carlton, had a hearing problem. I took him to the Mayo Clinic, and the three-day exam showed his hearing was normal. The doctor suggested he be tested by the psychology department. We returned the next weekend for a two-day exam, after which another doctor assured us that everything was normal. (He did say that Carlton was a bright child and was probably not responding to us because his mind was on something else.) We never received a bill for any of the five days at the clinic.

21

Opal's Toothache
The Wonders of Acupuncture

> The power that made the body can heal the body.
> *Ancient Proverb*

Acupuncture has always fascinated me. I started learning about the intricacies of this ancient healing art by taking a couple of weekend classes taught by freelance instructors. Then in 1973, after completing a three-hundred-hour acupuncture course conducted by the Columbia College of Chiropractic in New York, I became a certified acupuncturist. American acupuncture was just in its infancy at that time.

The Columbia course was directed by Dr. Richard Yennie, a highly respected acupuncturist and chiropractor. He had grown up in Japan, where his father worked as a member of the U.S. diplomatic service, and studied Japanese health-care methods and acupuncture. Returning to the states at the start of World War II, he attended chiropractic college to master yet another form of nonmedical healing. His superb credentials certainly made him qualified to teach acupuncture to chiropractors. He also invited renowned instructors from throughout Asia to participate as guest lecturers. The course was excellent.

I learned that acupuncture dates back nearly four thousand years, originating in China, and is used to treat numerous health problems. Its basis is strictly philosophical; Western science has no explanation for how or why it works. According to ancient oriental theories, an internal force or energy, *chi*, travels through fourteen distinct pathways, or *meridians*, similar to the nerves and blood vessels that cover the body. One meridian travels along the spine (the *governing vessel*); another along the midline of the abdomen (the *conception vessel*); and each of the remaining twelve corresponds to a different organ. The organ meridians fall into one of two groups, the *yin* and *yang*. The six yin meridians are heart, lungs, liver, kidney, spleen, and the *pericardium* (the sac surrounding the heart); and the six yang meridians are stomach, gall bladder, bladder, small intestine, large intestine, and one called the *triple-heater*. (This isn't actually an organ; instead, it can be viewed as the metabolism, corresponding to three heat-generating areas: the head and neck area, the chest above the diaphragm, and the lower abdomen below the diaphragm.)

Modern medical science teaches us that the *autonomic* branch of the nervous system regulates the body's internal organs and is divided into two parts: the *sympathetic system* and the *parasympathetic system*. These systems perform opposite actions, and all organs contain nerves from both. Sympathetic nerves act to speed up sympathetic-dominated organs, and parasympathetic nerves slow them down. Likewise, parasympathetic nerves accelerate parasympathetic-dominated organs, and sympathetic nerves sedate them.

The early Chinese seemed to be aware of this complex relationship. They had grouped together all of the sympathetic-dominated organs (yin) and all of the parasympathetic-dominated ones (yang). They had learned, as their modern counterparts had, that during periods of high stress, the body relies primarily on the yin organs. When confronted with a dangerous "fight or flight" situation, an individual needs his yin (sympathetic-dominated) organs to function at peak performance: The heart needs to beat faster, supplying more blood to the muscles used for fighting or fleeing; the lungs must absorb more oxygen for the strenuous activity; the increased waste from this action forces the liver and kidneys to accelerate their functions to eliminate it; and the spleen, which manufactures blood cells, is also kicked into high gear.

At the same time, the body can't afford to channel any energy into digestion, shutting down the yang (parasympathetic-dominated) organs (stomach, bladder, gall bladder, small intestine, and bowel). If the circumstances are severe enough, sometimes the energy stops completely, resulting in a "knot in the stomach" or even a loss of bladder or bowel control.

So how did they determine which organs are yin and which are yang? According to ancient Chinese religion, a severed body part had to be preserved and buried with the rest of the body, or the person would have to live in heaven without it. Consequently, the original doctors of acupuncture were not doing research on cadavers four thousand years ago. By what means, then, did they develop such a complex healing system two thousand years before the time of Christ? No one knows.

Nevertheless, over several centuries, the early Chinese managed to identify 365 specific points distributed along the meridian lines that are effective treatment areas. (Twelve organ meridians and twelve months in the year; 365 points and 365 days in the year—an intriguing relationship.) An acupuncturist inserts fine needles (about the thickness of horsehair) into these points, stimulating the chi in some areas, while reducing it in others. In this way, acupuncture restores an energetic balance to the body. The Chinese believe that pain and illness are caused by an absence of free-flowing chi, and when balance is achieved, healing can occur. The needles are inserted from a quarter inch to a full inch in depth and cause little to no discomfort for the patient.

Throughout my training, I repeatedly asked how and why this process worked, and I always received the same answer, "Don't ask. It just does."

Indeed, the instructors provided several demonstrations to prove the veracity and effectiveness of acupuncture. Dr. Wong, a Chinese acupuncturist from Hong Kong, showed us a particularly memorable point called *Zhong Ji*, or *Conception Vessel 3* (CV3), a point located midline, approximately one inch above the place where the pubic bones meet. He requested the young woman who sat outside the lecture room taking attendance to help with the demonstration. He told her to lie face up on the banquet-size table at the front of the class, and then inserted a needle through her clothing and into CV3. Seconds later, she let out a startled gasp and began to blush. Dr. Wong explained to the class that she'd just experienced an orgasm. Once we all stopped laughing, we sat there stunned—and impressed.

Near the end of the course, I began to realize that acupuncture and chiropractic share many similarities. Just as acupuncture needles can open up a blocked energy path, so can an adjustment remove an impediment to normal nerve flow. And in both healing methods, once the practitioner eliminates the restrictions, the body is allowed to heal itself.

This revelation and the dramatic results I witnessed made me keen on incorporating acupuncture into my practice. Shortly after I received my certification, Opal, a beauty operator, came to see me for her regular appointment. As I was working on her back, she asked, "I've got this awful toothache. Can chiropractic do anything for it?"

"No, unfortunately, dentistry is outside the realm of chiropractic," I said, but then I had a thought. "You know, acupuncture just might give you some relief until you can get to a dentist." I checked my reference book to find the proper points.

I read that stimulating the *He Gu,* or *Large Intestine 4* (LI4), point, the fourth point on the large intestine meridian, would relieve a toothache in the lower jaw, while *Nei Ting,* the forty-fourth point on the stomach meridian (ST44), would help an upper jaw toothache.

"Show me where the pain is," I said, and Opal opened her mouth and put her finger on the lower right molar area.

The LI4 point, located on the back of both hands, is easily identified: Place either hand flat on the table top and press your thumb as close to the rest of the hand as possible. LI4 sits at the end of the wrinkle that forms between the thumb and the hand. I inserted the needle into that spot on Opal's right hand—to treat the right side of her lower jaw—and left it in for several minutes to sedate the toothache. (To stimulate the area, I would have left it in for only seven seconds.)

After I removed the needle, Opal's eyes widened in surprise. "Gosh, the pain is almost completely gone—already," she said. "It really works."

Acupuncture's popularity in the United States has grown at an amazing rate over the past thirty years. Some medical schools have even begun to include acupuncture as part of their curriculum. I have used acupuncture as an ancillary feature in my practice, mostly relying on it as an effective pain reliever. Beyond that, this powerful healing technique can remedy acute or chronic illnesses, boost the body's recuperative powers, and strengthen the immune system. Without side effects when administered by a certified practitioner, acupuncture can help treat a wide variety of conditions, ranging from respiratory disorders to gynecological complaints. And it is safe: Regulated by the U.S. Food and Drug Administration (FDA), needles are individually wrapped, sterilized, disposable, and never reused, so there is no danger of contamination.

22

Ursula and the Pill
A Little Bit of Humor

Nature has never been wrong, nor has she changed her rules, since the world began.
Howard Loomis, D.C.

Ursula worked as a clerk behind the counter at the post office in southeast Boulder. Whenever I stopped there, I'd prefer Ursula to help me, knowing her playful, outgoing manner would brighten my day. On one particular morning, her pale face and strained expression told me she wasn't feeling well. I asked her what was wrong. "Oh, it's one of my migraines," she muttered, "and I really shouldn't be working. I could take a sick day, but we're already shorthanded."

I generally don't blow my own horn, yet I couldn't leave her in such distress. "You know, Ursula, I'm a chiropractor, and I treat many patients with migraines. Spinal adjustments can definitely ease your symptoms." Since several people were still waiting in line, I kept it brief. I gave her my card, picked up the rolls of stamps, and proceeded to the office.

Later that morning, I overheard my receptionist scheduling a new patient for the noon hour. At twelve o'clock, I found Ursula sitting in an examination room, bent over, her head in her hands. "I've tried everything . . . to get rid of . . . these migraines," she said, barely above a whisper, "but, nothing works . . . I've never been to a chiropractor before . . . I'll do anything . . . I'm desperate."

I figured she wasn't the least bit interested in a long-winded lecture on the relationship between neck misalignments and headaches. Ursula needed relief and she needed it immediately. I quickly examined her and took the necessary x-rays. After developing and reviewing the films, I adjusted her *atlas* (the top neck vertebra) and the *axis* (the second vertebra just below the atlas). Then I turned off the lights and instructed her to lie quietly. When I stepped back into the room a few minutes later, I asked her how she felt. She smiled. "My headache is almost completely gone," she said.

I told her to sit up slowly. "Ursula, are you taking birth control pills?"

She looked puzzled "Yes, I am. Why do you ask?"

"Sometimes a migraine headache can be a side effect of the pill. The body uses vitamin B-6, or *pyridoxine*, to detoxify the pill's hormone substances. This vitamin also controls the blood vessels that supply the brain. If the body's B-6 reservoir is depleted to offset the pill's effects, nothing is left over to properly regulate the brain's blood supply. As a result, you can develop a migraine headache."

Ursula rose from the adjusting table and thanked me. She made an appointment for the following day just in case her headache returned.

When I saw Ursula the next morning, her face glowed. "I feel like a million bucks!" she cried. She had been thinking about our conversation and asked me questions about chiropractic and bionutrition. After talking a half hour or so, Ursula became a believer in the natural approach to healing—namely, finding the cause and fixing it, rather than merely treating the symptoms.

To replace the vitamin B-6 she was losing with birth control pills, I gave her a bottle of B-6 supplements to take with meals. I informed her that all B vitamins are water soluble and must be consumed daily because they can't be stored in the body. Normally, these vitamins should be taken together, but certain conditions or deficiencies, like Ursula's, demanded two to three times more of one B vitamin than another. Although most foods contain small amounts of B-6, Ursula needed a much larger amount to offset the pill's effects.

About three weeks later, Ursula's name appeared again in the appointment book. "How are you feeling today?" I asked, greeting her in an adjusting room.

She started grinning. "I'm actually feeling great. I just had to come in and tell you what happened. Yesterday, I went to my gynecologist for my annual pap smear. Everything went fine, and while I was there, I asked him, 'Is it true that a woman can lose vitamin B-6 while she's on the pill?' And he said, 'Yes, there's some evidence supporting that possibility.'"

Ursula's grin grew wider. "So I asked him, 'If that's true, why don't you tell women to take extra B-6 when you give them prescriptions for the pill?'" She was laughing now. "And can you guess what he said?" I couldn't, but judging from her expression, I knew the punch line was going to be good. "He said, 'Oh, we couldn't do that because we don't know the side effects of B-6.'"

I laughed along with her. It's funny and so true. Without hesitating, many physicians will prescribe a drug that has numerous side effects, some of which are highly detrimental. They seldom, if at all, delve into nature's safe, bountiful resources. Amazing.

23

Pesky Nail Fungus
A Different Approach

> Seeing medical experts like Dr Andrew Weil and Dr. Deepak Chopra embrace and promote alternative, holistic healing tells me that the essence of what chiropractic has been for 110 years is permeating mainstream health care.
>
> *Michael Ameli*
> President, Alumni Association
> Northwestern University of Health Sciences, 2004

JOE'S TOENAIL FUNGUS

Exactly nine miles west of Hector lies a small town called Bird Island. According to its chamber of commerce, no other place in the entire world shares this unique name. Joe grew up there, and after his high school graduation in 1949, he joined the U.S. Marines, ready to perform his patriotic duty. Upon completion of basic training, the corps shipped him overseas to do battle in Korea.

Like many combat soldiers who served before him, Joe learned quickly that "war is hell." His unit sloshed through rice paddies in the summer months and climbed the mountainous slopes in the biting cold of the Korean winters. Because the battle lines shifted rapidly up and down the peninsula, the men remained in the field for many months at a time without fresh supplies. Consequently, they had to make do with whatever they had. Often, several days and even weeks passed before Joe could remove his shoes, much less change his socks. This highly unsanitary condition plus the perpetual wading through rivers and swamps led to the development of a fungal infection in Joe's toenails. Reproducing via spores, fungi thrive in warm, moist environments and once embedded are very difficult to eliminate. Even when Joe moved to drier ground, he still couldn't avoid recontamination since his socks had already become a constant source of reinfection.

After his discharge, Joe returned home to Bird Island. The fungus continued to erode the flesh around his toenails, troubling him nonstop. As the fungus multiplied, it built up a hard *keratinous* (nail-like) accumulation under the nail and extensively deformed the nail bed. The medical doctors at the marine discharge center had given him a prescription for an antifungal cream to rub into the tissues. Although it gradually cleared up the condition, the fungus always managed to reappear.

Joe visited his local physician who changed the medication, but unfortunately it produced the same disappointing results. He sensed that the problem was actually under the toenails; yet, even with Q-tips, Joe couldn't apply the cream all the way up under the nail to kill off the entire fungus. He then tried clipping his toenails as short as possible to remove any refuge for the fungus to hide. No success. Another physician advised soaking his feet in a special medicated solution, but the surface tension of the liquid precluded its completely reaching under the nail. Nothing made a lasting difference. Eventually, the insidious fungus would recur.

Joe had joined the American Legion Post in his hometown and regularly attended the monthly meetings. On one occasion, when his feet felt especially uncomfortable, he quietly slipped off his shoes. A Legion buddy sitting next to him noticed. "What's wrong?" he asked.

"It's that damn jungle rot I picked up in Korea—sure wish I could get rid of the damn thing."

"You know, I go to Dr. Rude, my chiropractor in Hector, for everything. He does a lot of other things besides crack my back. He uses electrical equipment and other instruments. Maybe he knows a different kind of treatment that would help. It wouldn't do any harm to give him a try. Go see if he can kill the fungus."

And that's what Joe did. He came to my office and shared his story. I asked him for details about the soaking solution he had been using. "It's a copper sulfate mixture," he said, "but it doesn't work much better than the salve."

From my chemistry classes, I had learned that copper could act as a fungicide. For it to be 100 percent effective, however, it had to fully penetrate the area and kill *all* fungi and spores to guard against any recontamination. It was crucial the liquid reach into all the tiny crevices to thoroughly destroy every trace.

I thought back to my chemical engineering classes at the University of Minnesota and remembered a significant fact: Copper can be electroplated (electrically extracted) from a copper electrolyte solution through the application of a direct electrical current. My *galvanic electrotherapy unit* generated a low-voltage direct current, primarily used for promoting healing when introduced into the body. With a little ingenuity, I could use this instrument and invent a method for transferring the copper ions into the skin and nails. Using a weak electrical current to transfer the ions of a medication into the body's tissues is a technique called *iontophoresis*. I had used it successfully in several other situations. Before applying it to Joe, though, I first had to determine the consequences of introducing additional copper into the body.

I described the ion-transfer procedure to Joe, explaining I'd need more time to research it. "Make an appointment for tomorrow," I said, "and bring the copper mixture. Also, because spores are probably hiding in your socks and shoes, bring along a new pair of each to prevent reinfection." Joe agreed and left looking encouraged.

Good health dictates that our tissues contain minute amounts of copper as well as other trace minerals. I dug out my biochemistry books and read that copper enhances the action of vitamin C and some of the B vitamins. Therefore, a small amount of extra copper would probably do no harm. I thumbed through the textbook from my physical therapy class at National College of Chiropractic and discovered a short section on iontophoresis. It reported that copper could be used as a fungicide using positive galvanic current. (Darn it! So much for my original idea. . . .)

When I saw Joe the following day, he was carrying a half-full quart bottle of the copper-sulfate liquid.

"You know, I'm not sure that'll be enough," I told him. "I'll call the local druggist and ask him to make up an additional gallon of the stuff. Please pick it up and we'll try it as soon as you get back."

After he returned, I pulled out a plastic dishpan and filled it with the blue solution. Both feet fit in the basin and were totally submerged. "This setup will work perfectly," I said. "By eliminating even the smallest exposed areas, we can avoid reinfection." I dropped the positive pad from the galvanic unit into the pan. To complete the electrical circuit, I thoroughly wet the negative pad and attached it firmly to his bare right arm. (Any place on the body will work.)

I switched on the instrument and slowly increased the voltage. Since copper is a positive ion, the negative pad (Joe's arm) attracted it and the positive pad (the solution) repelled it. The tissues of his feet actually sucked up the copper sulfate. "Let me know if you begin to feel any discomfort," I said.

It wasn't long before he mentioned he felt some tingling. I immediately stopped turning up the voltage.

"Can you tolerate that level?" I asked.

"Yeah, it's okay right there."

We talked about his war exploits and local issues for about five minutes. Then I turned off the machine, dried his feet, and poured the solution back into the gallon container.

"Come back tomorrow," I said. "I'd like to check your feet. I'll keep the jug here."

The next day he greeted me with good news. "I think it's working. I went to the Legion meeting last night and my feet didn't bother me as much."

I reconnected the galvanic unit, and again Joe dunked his feet into the blue liquid. Everything proceeded as it had the day before, and again he left after making an appointment for the next day.

The possibility of overdosing him with copper still concerned me, particularly with daily treatments. Serious side effects could rear their ugly heads. I returned to my books for help and read an article about a researcher who had orally administered copper and found that a heavy dose caused stomachaches. When I saw Joe the following day, I asked him if he'd been feeling abnormal in any way.

"No, not at all," he said, shaking his head. "In fact, I'm really pleased—my feet have improved so much after only two treatments. They feel better now than they did before I left the marines." I repeated the protocol and decided to forego scheduling any appointments for the upcoming weekend.

On Monday I carefully examined Joe's feet. His blue-tinged toenails were clearly less disfigured than they had been a week earlier. "Since I was feeling a lot better," he said, "I tried to remove some of the crusty stuff that was growing under the nail. They look pretty good, don't they?"

I administered another dose of the copper-sulfate and suggested he come back on Thursday. One dilemma persisted: What constituted enough? I was exploring new vistas and had no idea when to stop. If I discontinued the treatment at this point, would the fungus recur as it had with all the other remedies? On the other hand, would I ultimately overdose him with copper?

After two additional treatments I told Joe, "I think we'll stop here. If the fungus reappears again, we'll know we quit too soon."

"If it comes back, I'll be back," he said and thanked me for helping him.

Close to three years later, as I was cleaning out the cupboard in the x-ray room, I found the gallon jug of copper sulfate solution. I had stored it in case Joe experienced a relapse, which apparently never happened. I didn't encounter another case of fungus until long after moving to Colorado.

OLLIE: ANOTHER KOREAN WAR VET

Over the years I've observed a trend among my patients. Nearly all of them seem very pleased with the outcome of the therapies I recommend. The majority are very grateful and return for spinal adjustments when necessary. A small percentage will refer their family members and friends. My favorites, of course, are the select few I call "bird dogs," the ones who seldom miss an opportunity to send someone my way—Joe's buddy at the Legion Post is a perfect example.

Ray, a local merchant and one of my Boulder patients, behaves the same way. An avid tennis player, he belongs to the racquet club at the Hilton Harvest House. One day he was scheduled to play Ollie, a retired U.S. Army colonel. Ollie explained he'd have to postpone the match because he had a sore toe and couldn't run. Ray immediately said, "Go across the street to my chiropractor, Dr. Rude. He takes care of just about everything, and I'm sure he can fix your toe."

FUNGUS/GOUT

Following his friend's advice, Ollie limped into my office. When I examined his feet, I found a badly swollen and inflamed big toe—it looked like an overgrown radish. My first thought was *gout*. Although fungus had also spread throughout his toenails, the ugly, red enlarged toe was certainly the cause of his limp.

"Ollie, this looks like gout to me—a blood test will let us know for sure. I'll call the lab and set up an appointment." When I returned to the exam room, I said, "They can see you at two this afternoon. By the way, how long have you had that fungus in your toenails?"

"I picked that up in Korea. My wife thinks it's horrible. I've learned to live with it and I guess she has too, since I've never found anything that will cure it."

Coincidentally, I was writing this chapter at that time, so I instructed my receptionist to give Ollie a copy. He appeared slightly confused, which was understandable. After all, here was a back doctor who examined his toe, ordered blood tests, and then handed him information on the treatment of another fellow's fungus.

On his way to the lab, Ollie stopped to see his medical doctor who confirmed the need for the test. And just as I had predicted, the results showed a very high *uric acid*, a positive sign for gout. Uric acid is a normal by-product of protein metabolism, and increased levels are generally associated with a high-purine diet: organ meats (liver, kidney, and sweetbreads), shellfish, brewer's yeast (beer), baker's yeast (baked goods and bread), anchovies, sardines, herring, mackerel, and alcohol. Gout is a form of arthritis caused by excess uric acid that crystallizes in the joints, usually in the joint of the first toe.

Ollie's M.D. prescribed the drug *colchicine*. This medication does not lower uric acid levels but works instead to reduce inflammation in the affected area. Because this drug's adverse reactions include muscular weakness, nausea, vomiting, diarrhea, hives, dermatitis, and hair loss, most people can't tolerate it. Although his symptoms abated within three weeks, Ollie was exposing himself to unnecessary risks.

I regret not discussing naturopathic remedies with Ollie. Fortunately, both conventional and alternative medicine agree that changes in diet and lifestyle are essential for healing gout. Health-care practitioners recommend eliminating uric acid–forming foods and consuming foods rich in potassium, such as bananas, beans, leafy green vegetables, and cherries—especially large quantities of cherry juice (unsweetened). Drinking plenty of water and maintaining a healthy body weight are always excellent ideas. In lieu of colchicine and its potential side effects, I suggest taking one-half teaspoon of potassium bicarbonate (*not* sodium bicarbonate) twice daily and the following Standard Process products: *Arginex* (three to nine tablets), *Comfrey*, *Pepsin*, and *E3*—a source of *allantoin*, a substance that aids in uric acid metabolism.

Soon after his gout cleared, Ollie's son, a chemical engineer, visited his dad over Father's Day weekend. Ollie described his experience at my office and shared the copy of "Joe's Toenail Fungus." His son's response sent Ollie back to me for treatment. " 'That's a very unique idea and it should work,' " he quoted his son.

We began the iontophoresis, and in a mere two weeks, the fungus was in check, thoroughly amazing Ollie. At his follow-up appointment a couple of weeks later, I saw no signs of fungus. And I was very pleased to discover that Ollie now believed in the effectiveness of alternative health care.

Erin's Fracture and Fingernails

During the time I was treating Ollie for his fungus, I met Erin, a vibrant young woman in her midtwenties. She came to my office wearing a cast on her right arm; she had fallen and fractured the *navicular* bone, one of the eight bones that make up the wrist. Her regular chiropractor, Dr. Duggan of Boulder, knew I had specialized equipment and recommended she consult me for treatments to speed the healing process.

I explained to Erin that this type of injury can be very serious. The fracture line crosses the artery supplying the navicular bone, cutting off the vital blood flow to part of the bone. As a result, the starved tissue can undergo irreversible damage and decompose, a condition called *necrosis*—sometimes, even gangrene can develop. I suggested we begin a *pulsed diathermy* regimen to increase circulation in her wrist and reduce the likelihood of any complications.

(Dating back to the early 1900s, diathermy is a form of physical therapy that induces heat in the body by means of controlled high frequency electromagnetic energy. Unfortunately, this modality could not be used on wounds because heat causes capillaries to dilate, leading to more bleeding. Then, in the early 1960s, experiments showed that *pulsed*, rather than continuous, energy can dramatically increase wound healing *without* producing heat. The Federal Drug Administration, or the FDA, later approved pulsed diathermy for healing orthopedic injuries.)

Erin quickly agreed with my recommendation. At one of her appointments she spotted Ollie sitting in the therapy room. "What's that guy doing with his feet in the blue water?" she asked.

I explained he was receiving therapy for his toenail fungus. "*I* have a fungus in my fingernails," she said. "Would that help me?" Her hand was covered by the cast, so I hadn't noticed the fungi in her nails. She must have been self-conscious about her other hand because she seemed to deliberately keep it out of sight.

"I'm pretty confident it would solve your problem."

"My doctor has me on *Lamisil*[*] right now. If that doesn't clear up the fungus, I'll come back here and try this. The cast would have to come off before I could soak my hands anyway."

And sure enough, I did see Erin about four weeks later. "My wrist healed really well," she told me. "My family doctor was surprised it happened so fast. He said I was very lucky because in many cases this kind of injury never improves—just like you said. Now, let's get started with the blue treatments to kill this ugly stuff on my nails. The medicine has helped some, but it gives me diarrhea and gas, and the fungus keeps hanging on."

Once we performed a series of the copper sulfate iontophoresis treatments, Erin's nails improved dramatically. Soon the fungus vanished altogether, and she no longer felt compelled to hide her hands.

---

[*]An antifungal pharmaceutical.

24

Chronic Motion Sickness
A Simple Remedy

> Our bones need a good source of calcium for strength, but it takes a corresponding amount of phosphorus for the calcium to do its job. Without phosphorus, calcium is largely washed out.
>
> *J. I. Rodale*
> Complete Book of Minerals

At seventy-one years old, Maude was one of my favorite senior citizens. She told me at her first visit, "I could have retired at sixty-five, but Mr. Stout, my boss at the shop, said, 'Maude, you can't retire. After all, I'm seventy-four and I'm *still* working. Besides, this place would fall apart without you.'" She was a real go-getter in the community, serving on two city committees, holding the office of precinct captain for her political party, and teaching Sunday school.

Maude had hurt her back helping Mr. Stout lift a heavy sink at his plumbing shop. Despite her injury, she maintained a positive attitude and even joked about her pain. "I guess when I buckled down to lift that sink, it was really my back that buckled."

Although not serious, her problem required a few visits to correct. If she had been younger, she probably would have responded more quickly.

At one appointment, Maude mentioned she had been a member of the Business and Professional Women's Organization for years. "They usually have their national conventions either on the east or west coast, and I've never had a chance to go," she said. "This year, though, it's up in Estes Park—in fact, it's coming up this weekend. I'd love to be there, but those twisty mountain roads always make me carsick, so I won't be going to that one either."

"Maude, do you mind if I make a suggestion?"

"Of course not, go right ahead."

"I give phosphorus to patients who suffer from motion sickness. It comes in a liquid form, and it's very easy to take. I use the Standard Process product called *Phosfood*. The recommended dosage is fifteen drops in eight ounces of water. I've had a lot of success with it."

"How does it taste?"

"Not bad. It's sour like fresh lemon juice without the lemon flavor. Would you like to try some?" Because phosphorus relieves nausea, I usually keep a bottle on hand to help unsettled stomachs. "It can't do you any harm," I assured her.

"Sure, I'm game."

I mixed up the solution and Maude drank it down. "You're right. It tastes okay."

"Take a bottle home with you and the night before the convention, take the fifteen drops as I've suggested and then again when you get up in the morning. I bet you'll be able to drive to Estes Park without a problem."

With a spring in her step and Phosfood in her hand, Maude left for the shop.

On the following Monday morning, my receptionist poked her head into the adjusting room. "Maude's on the phone," she said, "and she wants to talk with you—says it's important."

I barely managed to squeeze out a hello before Maude jumped in. "I made it all the way up to Estes and didn't feel the least bit carsick!" She was shouting so loudly I had to move the phone away from my ear. "It sure was nice to be able to ride through the mountains again. I'll tell you more at my appointment tomorrow."

Her high spirits were contagious, and as I returned to my patient, I felt thrilled knowing I had helped someone fulfill a longtime dream.

When I saw her the next day, Maude shone with excitement about the convention and her trip to the mountains. "Tell me about this magical phosphorus. How does it stop motion sickness?"

"Most likely because phosphorus lowers the viscosity, or stickiness, of blood—and probably all body fluids—which helps increase circulation and relieve the nausea."

I directed Maude to lie face down on the adjusting table and then began palpating her spine to check for misalignments.

"In general," I said, "nutritionists don't seem to pay much attention to phosphorus, yet it's the second most abundant mineral in our bodies, the first being calcium. Bone is actually the *phosphate* salts of calcium and magnesium. When bone breaks down, as in osteoporosis, not only is calcium depleted but phosphorus is depleted as well."

"You mean I should be taking phosphorus along with calcium to prevent osteoporosis?"

"Yes, it's a good idea. According to a study conducted by the National Institute of Dental Research at the Massachusetts Institute of Technology, a phosphorus deficiency can cause dental cavities. Considering bones and teeth are approximately the same in composition, I've often thought that adding phosphorus to the diet would treat osteoporosis. You have to remember, though, that the body contains twice as much calcium as phosphorus, so it's important to maintain that ratio."

I told Maude her back was improving and started adjusting the few subluxations I'd found.

"Now, another type of phosphate within the body is adenosine tri*phosphate*, or ATP," I continued. "This chemical helps our bodies produce energy by converting sugar into carbon dioxide and water. And the brain is composed of *phospholipid*s, another form of phosphorus that is attached to fatty molecules."

I completed the final adjustment. "Maude, we're done now, but you lie there for a minute and rest." I pulled up a chair and sat down.

"There's even more to the story: Phosphorus can eliminate joint stiffness, especially the kind you may have in the morning that disappears once you move around. And it's also a good remedy for excess hydrochloric acid in the stomach. Incidentally, antacids reduce the body's phosphorus levels and can lead to bone loss. I sometimes wonder about the relationship between osteoporosis and a high intake of antacids."

"I've taken my share of antacids—I get a sour stomach a lot. Could that be the reason why I get carsick? I didn't have the problem when I was younger, and I didn't have stomach trouble either."

"Could be you've answered your own question."

"Maybe I should take phosphorus on a regular basis. I understand how it works with calcium, and especially at my age, I have to watch out for osteoporosis. Many of the things you mentioned fit my case. What do you think?" She sat up on the table.

"Actually, I don't recommend that for you. Phosphorus levels can change with your diet and will even fluctuate throughout the day depending on what you're eating. It's in many foods—meat, wheat germ, sunflower seeds, soy products, eggs, and brewer's yeast. Too much can have harmful side effects, like changes in blood pressure, or a large increase in the metabolism or heartbeat, particularly when the thyroid isn't functioning properly. Also, pregnant women in their last trimester shouldn't take phosphorus, but then you don't have to worry about that, do you?" I smiled.* "I suggest we run a blood test to determine your actual calcium and phosphorus levels. And it would be wise to do a complete physical. If your blood pressure and heart rate are on the low side, you just might have a phosphorus deficiency."

Maude turned into a biochemistry patient instead of just a chiropractic one with a pain in the back. Her blood tests showed she would indeed benefit from a phosphorus supplement.

I addressed all of Maude's health concerns over the next few years. I not only solved her motion sickness but also helped prevent osteoporosis and other age-related problems. Mr. Stout *did* eventually retire and so did Maude. She moved to California to live out her life near her son.

---

*As I explained, calcium phosphate is one of the main ingredients in bones—it is the phosphate portion that strengthens and hardens them. During the last trimester of pregnancy, the mother's bones and teeth supply the calcium needed for the development of the fetus's bones. Because their bones don't need to be strong in the womb, just the calcium is extracted from the mother. Consequently, her own calcium level drops relative to that of phosphorus. Taking additional phosphorus at this time would further disrupt the calcium/phosphate balance.

25

Harry's Hay Fever
Secondary Benefits

> Look to the spine for the cause of disease.
> *Hippocrates*
> *Father of Medicine, (460–370 B.C.)*

Although most southern Minnesota residents are not surprised by the occasional rip-snortin' blizzard, nothing had prepared me for the severe one that raged all night in the middle of January 1954. The weatherman had predicted some snow and possible gusty winds in the rural areas, but he clearly had underestimated the power of the storm.

When I awoke to a bleak white landscape stretched as far as the eye could see, I decided to stay home and not risk driving to the office. Experience had taught me that Minnesota wind could whip up the snow, making frozen snowbanks a man could easily walk over, while a car would sink and become lodged. Besides, I heard on the radio that the roads were impassable.

Toward noon, the phone rang.

"Dr. Rude? This is Glenda Brennan—Rudy Nester told me to call you. I couldn't reach you at the clinic. I thought you might still be at home." She was breathing hard. "We've got an emergency. Ed—my husband—got hurt. Outside. Don't know how long he was stuck out there. He's in a lot of pain. Rudy and his buddy Al are taking him to your office."

"Easy—slow down. Can you tell me what happened?" I'd heard of "Big Ed" Brennan. I knew he and his wife owned a large dairy farm located a good half mile from the county road.

She took a deep breath and let it out. "Well, no, I can't tell you *exactly*. I do know Ed left the house real early to plow the driveway so he could haul the milk to town. Then a little while later, I happened to look out the window and all I saw was the tractor—no Ed. I got a bad feeling so I jumped in the car and drove down the driveway. I found him flat on his back, mumbling something about flying off the tractor. He's way too large for me to handle—I had to call our neighbor Rudy."

Rudy, his brother, Lester, and his two sisters, Clara and Emma, had been my parents' patients for years. My mom and dad had a home-office combination, and I remembered back when I was in junior high that the Nestors started coming for their regular adjustments. Naturally, Rudy's first thought was to take Big Ed to the chiropractor.

"How are they going to make it into town?"

"Well, Rudy and Al loaded him onto a bobsled—they just left. I sure hope you can help my Ed. I'm real worried he has frostbite—good Lord, it must be close to twenty below out there."

I peered out at the deep snow. "I'll be waiting for them," I said, trying to sound more confident than I really felt.

Knowing the Brennan farm sat about seven miles northwest of Hector, I assumed the trip would take them awhile (although with a bobsled, they might actually be waiting for *me*). I managed to get my car down the driveway and headed south toward the office. After about two blocks, a huge drift stopped me, forcing me to drive east to Main Street, which had been recently plowed. I turned south on Main and eventually parked at a gas station within half a block of my office. All the roads I normally used were completely buried in mountains of snow.

At the office, I waited for the bobsled to arrive. Since heat would be the number-one priority for Ed, I turned up the thermostat and wheeled the *diathermy unit* into the adjusting room. The electromagnetic energy from this device produces internal heat as it passes through the body—just as a toaster element heats up due to the resistance in the wire. Ed wouldn't actually feel the transfer of energy, but he'd notice he was slowly warming up.

Soon I saw a team of horses dragging an old bobsled down the street. I held the door open while Rudy and Al carried Big Ed into the adjusting room, and I directed them to lay him on the exam table. I saw immediately how he'd earned his nickname—he must have been nearly six and a half feet tall, probably over three hundred pounds, and very easily could have been a tackle for the Minnesota Vikings in his younger days. Certainly no match for his wife.

Ed was much too cold for me to even consider beginning an examination or any form of treatment. I checked him for signs of frostbite, found none, and then attached the diathermy unit to him, with one end on his buttocks and the other over his shoulders. In this way, the diathermy energy could pass through most of his body, quickly warming him.

Waiting for Ed to recover, I asked Rudy and Al if they knew what had happened.

"Well, what we figure is this," Rudy began. "The Brennans have to deliver the milk on time to avoid spoilage. And normally Ed has no trouble fighting the snow. He's got this special oversized scooper rigged to his tractor for loadin' and haulin' the piles of manure his cows leave behind. During the winter, this scooper comes in real handy for clearing a path down his driveway. He usually races down the driveway and uses it to blast through the drifts. So this morning after the storm, Ed went out to the machine shed and fired up the tractor. Al and I guess something went wrong after that."

Ed began to move. "You've got it right," he said, his lips still slightly blue. "I rammed into this hard-packed snow pile—it must have been six feet tall—as solid as concrete. It stopped the tractor dead in its tracks and threw me flying into the air. I landed smack on my back. I couldn't stand up or roll over or even crawl—every time I moved, this burning pain shot down my back and leg. Glenda covered me with lots of blankets and told me Rudy was coming over to help. But, damn, was I gettin' cold." He winced from the pain.

"I knew I'd be facing some tough snowdrifts," Rudy said, "so I pulled out an old bobsled, a leftover from my dad's day back when he homesteaded our farm. I needed some horses to haul Ed, but I'd replaced all of mine with tractors. Then I remembered Al Smoot a couple miles north—he used to have a team."

"Yeah, Rudy called me," Al chimed in. "When he explained how serious things were, I told him I'd go right out and hitch up the team. Said I'd hurry and make it to his place inside an hour—which I think I did."

Groaning, Ed turned to his friends. "Thanks, guys. . . . I really owe you for saving my life."

The diathermy had done its trick, and I started to examine Ed's back by palpating his spine. Since this was his first chiropractic visit, I carefully explained everything I was doing. His severe pain prevented him from moving to the x-ray room, so I told him I'd perform some preliminary massage and tissue work. When his muscles finally relaxed, I encouraged him to sit up, but immediately his back went into spasm. I had to resume the massage to coax his muscles to relax—his back musculature was one gigantic spasm.

"Ed, I've decided to forgo x-rays," I said. "I'll do just a mild chiropractic adjustment based on the physical exam, although you will need an x-ray as soon as you can stand erect." I debated about mentioning that he would hear a popping sound with the adjustment, concerned that any apprehension would cause him to tighten up again. Being honest with my patients is important to me, but this time I chose discretion instead and said nothing.

After waiting for him to relax completely, I adjusted his back. I felt and heard the release as the thrust changed the deviant vertebra's position to a more normal one. Startled, Ed flew off the table and stood with his fists raised, ready to fight his attacker.

"Hey, whoa, Ed!" I yelled, putting my hands out. "Aren't you feeling *better*?"

"Huh? Better?" He slowly lowered his arms as a smile spread across his broad face. "Yeah, it *is* better. I still hurt, but the sharp pain is gone."

"You'll be stiff and sore," I explained, "although if you stay warm and get a good night's rest, you should be able to come back tomorrow. You need an x-ray and some additional treatment because you have seriously injured your back muscles and ligaments. It'll take time to heal."

Rudy and Al helped Ed back to the bobsled, and they headed home.

The next day, Ed drove his own car and walked into the office by himself. Curious about chiropractic and how it had given him such instant relief, Ed asked several questions about his condition. We talked as I reexamined him and took x-rays.

In those days, the standard chiropractic x-ray film was a full-spine picture, measuring fourteen by thirty-six inches. It provided an excellent overall view of the patient's spine, helping the doctor point out the exact cause of the problem. When research revealed in the 1960s that this procedure exposed the patient to unnecessary, dangerous amounts of radiation, the protocol changed. Now, only x-rays of the problem area are taken.

After showing the films to Ed, I outlined a series of adjustments to correct his injury. He conscientiously kept all his appointments.

At one visit, I checked all the original subluxations and announced, "Ed, I've got really good news for you. Everything checks out fine, so I won't be adjusting you today. Make an appointment for next week, and I'll examine you again. Let's hope there's no change."

And there wasn't. "I have more good news this time, Ed. Since your back is still okay, I don't think you'll need any more adjustments. If the problem ever returns, you'll know what to do."

"Gee, thanks," he said, shaking my hand in his massive one. "Good thing Rudy Nester brought me here. I never would have thought of going to a chiropractor."

That was actually the last time I treated Ed. A few years later, though, his name popped up while I was consulting with a new patient, Harry Hawn. I was reviewing Harry's paperwork and noticed he had written *hay fever* next to "chief complaint," and *none* next to "previous chiropractic care." That's odd, I thought. Although hay fever responds favorably to spinal adjustments, most people wouldn't think about consulting a chiropractor unless they'd already had some success with a chiropractor elsewhere.

"How long have you suffered from hay fever?" I asked during the initial consultation.

"All my life—at least as far back as I can remember. It was better when I was a kid, but then I didn't have to go out into the fields where all the pollen was."

"Why did you choose to see me about your problem?"

"Well, it wasn't *my* idea. It was really my boss who wanted me to come here." Despite his obvious skepticism, he evidently thought he needed to obey his employer.

"And who do you work for?" I wondered which patient had made such an unusual referral.

"Big Ed Brennan," he said and sneezed. "He hired me last fall. I help do most everything—milking, feeding the cows, cleaning the barns, hauling the manure." He sneezed again and blew his nose into a big red bandanna. "Since this spring, when we cut the hay for the first time, I've been having all kinds of problems—eyes watering, nose running. Gosh, sometimes, I can hardly breathe. Ed said you cured his hay fever and it never came back. If you can do that for me, I'd be forever thankful."

"But when I saw Ed, he had a very bad *back* condition. I didn't treat him for hay fever. He never said anything about it." I thought back to his x-rays. Those large films were actually worth a king's ransom. I remembered spotting a severe *cervical* (neck) subluxation that I had also corrected while treating him for his lower back injury. Nerves in the upper neck area can influence sinus, hay fever, and throat conditions. "Do me a favor, Harry. Please tell Ed to stop by my office when he comes to town. I'd really like to talk with him about his hay fever."

After palpating Harry's spine and taking x-rays, I discovered he had a cervical subluxation similar to his boss's. I recommended a course of adjustments, and in about three weeks, his hay fever was under control. Less than a month after that, his condition had completely cleared.

We were nearing the end of summer when my receptionist told me Ed Brennan was in the waiting room. Eager to talk with him, I modified a couple of appointments to open up some time.

We visited a short while about his back injury, and he assured me it hadn't bothered him since the last time he'd seen me.

"You know, Ed, your hired hand, Harry Hawn, saw me for his hay fever. He said you'd told him I treated *your* hay fever. I didn't even know you'd been suffering with it."

"Well, you sure cured me. Ever since I was twelve years old, I'd come down with hay fever every time the fields were blooming. But once you took care of my back four years ago, I stopped having trouble. You're the only doctor I've been to, so you must have done it when you popped my neck and back."

"That makes a lot of sense. You see, there are four nerves in the neck area—"

"Look, Doc, I really don't care why it worked. I just know you fixed me, and I'm not miserable anymore. If I have problems again, I'll be back."

And as far as I know, neither Ed nor Harry suffered another hay fever attack. Isn't chiropractic wonderful?

26

Evelyn's Calcific Bursitis
Chemistry Comes to the Rescue

> A healthy body is the guest chamber of the soul. A sick body, its prison.
>
> *Sir Francis Bacon*
> *(1561–1626)*

My family and I moved from Hector, Minnesota, to Boulder, Colorado, in mid-December 1969. Because it happened during the winter and so close to the holidays, the move was especially stressful. Fortunately, our longtime friends Jean and Jack Ray, who were already Boulder residents, eased our transition. They greeted us with a warm welcome along with an invitation to join them for Christmas dinner.

We had known the Rays for several years. Jean had been Shirley's roommate at Gustavus Adolphus College in St. Peter, Minnesota, and after Jack's graduation from Mankato State College, Shirley and I attended the Rays' wedding. (I recall vividly that someone had smeared limburger cheese all over their honeymoon car.) They subsequently had four children—three sons and a daughter. Back in 1969, the two older, athletic boys, John and Tom, played Little League baseball and were avid skiers. Their younger brother, Jimmy, was more interested in art than sports and consequently received considerable taunting from his older siblings. Jane, the youngest and a three-year-old then, was a cute, fiery-haired little miss who worked hard to keep up with her older brothers. It was difficult to imagine that both Jimmy and Jane would later become chiropractors. Although I never actually discussed my profession with them, I'd like to think that I influenced them in a positive way.

A staunch believer in natural healing methods, Jean watched her family's diet and always prepared healthy, nourishing meals. She insisted everyone consume adequate vitamins and minerals. And when it came to treating illnesses, her first stop was at the chiropractor's. Only if he could not resolve the problem with natural methods would she consult a medical physician. The Rays had been going to Dr. Matt Bartol, a former classmate of mine at National Chiropractic College. After his relocation out of the Boulder area, I became their family doctor.

Jean gladly referred her friend Evelyn Keith to my new clinic. Even though Evelyn was hesitant about visiting a chiropractor, her persistent shoulder pain pushed her to seek alternative care. At the initial consultation, I met an attractive fifty-three-year-old woman who appeared to be in her early forties, thanks to an excellent lifelong exercise program.

"About six months ago," she began, "I fell really hard on my left shoulder during a tennis match. My family physician took x-rays and assured me it wasn't broken or dislocated. 'Just wait for that bad bruise to heal,' he said. Since then I haven't been able to raise my arm above shoulder level—see?" She winced as she tried to show me.

I started the physical exam by palpating the soft region surrounding her shoulder joint. When I applied pressure about four inches below the top of her shoulder, the pain made Evelyn groan and pull away. I then tested her arm's range of motion and saw that extreme discomfort in every direction clearly restricted her movement.

I suggested taking an x-ray. The films taken in the emergency room at the time of her accident showed no apparent abnormalities. The new x-ray I developed exposed the culprit: Embedded in the soft tissue of the shoulder, just to the side of the *humerus* (upper arm bone), I observed a white spot about the size of a pinto bean. Its rim was not clearly demarcated, making it look like a small fuzzy ball of cotton.

"Evelyn, I've discovered the cause of your pain. You've got a condition known as *calcific bursitis*."

"Gee, what's that? I *am* familiar with bursitis, but I've never heard of *calcific* bursitis before."

CALCIFIC BURSITIS

"Well, a *bursa* is a fluid-filled sac that's found in many joints of the body. It acts as a cushion between the bones and the muscles or tendons, and also facilitates movement by lowering the friction between a joint and the surrounding tissue. *Bursitis* is an inflammation of the bursa, caused by either trauma or repeated physical activity. Your fall injured the bursa in your left shoulder, leading to the development of bursitis there."

"Uh-huh, I thought it was something like that. Now, what about the calcific part?"

"Well, that's a lot more complicated." I went on to explain that bruising and healing generally follow an injury like hers. A bruise is formed by the blood that leaks out of damaged capillaries, and as healing progresses, the blood usually undergoes five distinct chemical changes: (1) The walls of the red blood cells break down, and the red, oxygenated *hemoglobin* (a protein substance) oozes out into the tissue. (2) Once the oxygen dissipates, the area turns a reddish-blue—this is the reason for the "black and blue" nature of a bruise. (3) The hemoglobin converts into *bilirubin* and becomes an orange-red. (4) The bilirubin gradually transforms into *biliverdin*, taking on a greenish hue. And (5) the biliverdin turns into *bilixanthin* and develops a yellow cast. As this whole process unfolds, some cells from each stage are picked up by normal circulation and travel back to the liver to become bile.

"In your case, however, a large quantity of blood had oozed into the bursa fluid, preventing it from experiencing the normal changes of a bruise. Iron—the main component of hemoglobin—is incompatible with the bursa's fluid. Your body viewed the iron as foreign matter and reacted by replacing it with a calcium molecule, which is the normal response in this kind of situation. Over a period of months, then, your body formed a small calcified mass in your left shoulder. Originally, you had restricted movement due to bursitis, but now it is the calcium deposit that's limiting you."

Evelyn looked bewildered. "You sure weren't kidding, were you? It's *very* complicated. But, is there anything you can *do* about it?"

"Yes. As a matter of fact, I just attended a seminar in Denver, led by two faculty members from Los Angeles Chiropractic College. Calcific bursitis was one of the subjects they discussed." Dr. Maynard

Lipe had described how *iontophoresis*[*] with iodine would thoroughly resolve this condition: The calcium deposit in the body could be removed by electroplating a negatively-charged iodine molecule into the affected region using current from a *galvanic unit* (this instrument's low-voltage direct current is typically used to promote healing when applied to the body). Iodine reacts with calcium and becomes calcium iodide, a substance that would easily dissolve in tissue fluids. Dr. Lipe had stressed the importance of using *organic* liquid iodine, warning us that regular synthetic on-the-shelf antiseptic iodine would be ineffective. Anabolic Laboratories of Irvine, California, is one of the few distributors of *Ioplex-a-dine*, an all-natural liquid iodine manufactured from seaweed.

Over a period of five weeks, we successfully eliminated the calcium deposit from Evelyn's shoulder. Her pain on movement disappeared and her full range of motion returned.

"Thank you so much," she told me. "I always had doubts about chiropractors and chiropractic but not anymore. I'm very glad I followed Jean's suggestion to come talk with you."

"It's really Jean you need to thank. I'm sure she'd appreciate it."

"I'll do that for sure. I'll be seeing her at church on Sunday."

Evelyn joined the growing list of advocates for natural, alternative healing. Like Jean, she referred several people to my office, and all of them responded well to chiropractic, nutritional, and physical therapies.

---

[*]The introduction of the ions of a medication into body tissues via a weak electrical current. See chapter 23 for a thorough discussion of this technique.

27

Ruby's Poor Old Back
Surgery Is Not the Only Answer

> Sickness is for those who do not know what to do about ill health.
>
> *Allen Stjernholm, D.C.*

For years Alice had suffered from stiff joints. Then in the early 1970s she learned that acupuncture might help her. She'd been reading a lot about it ever since President Nixon traveled to China in 1972. While the whole world watched, one of the journalists in Nixon's entourage had undergone an emergency appendectomy, and the Chinese physicians used acupuncture as the only anesthetic. Impressed, the president initiated an exchange program between medical practitioners in the two countries, sparking a growing fascination in the West for this ancient healing art.

After hearing about an acupuncturist in Portland, Oregon, who might help her condition, Alice left her home in Dodge City, Kansas, and started the long drive out to consult with him. For the first night of her journey, she stayed at her sister June's in Arvada, Colorado, a northern suburb of Denver. Before dinner, the two women went shopping at the Health Food Cottage, where June introduced her sister to Rita, the owner. During the conversation, Alice mentioned she had arthritis and was heading to Oregon for acupuncture treatments.

"Gosh, you don't have to go all that way," Rita told her. "I go to a chiropractor in Boulder, just fourteen miles north on the turnpike. He's used acupuncture on me—he knows a lot about it."

That's how I came to know and treat Alice. I helped ease her arthritis with acupuncture, nutrition, and chiropractic adjustments.

On one trip to Boulder, Alice brought along her other sister, Ruby. They had driven more than four hundred miles to find out if I could treat her chronic low-back condition and a more recent neck complaint.

I reviewed Ruby's history and discovered she had been suffering from lower back problems for more than twenty years, beginning with an overlifting injury. After putting up with the pain for two years, she consulted an orthopedic surgeon who determined that the *disk* between L5 (the lowest lumbar vertebra) and S1 (the first sacral vertebra) had ruptured. In the space between each vertebra is a spongy cushion—a disk—that has a fibrous outer layer protecting a softer gel-like center. If a disk ruptures, a part of this gel can be displaced, putting painful pressure on a spinal nerve or on the spinal cord. Ruby's surgeon recommended that it be removed, allowing the two vertebrae to eventually fuse together. She agreed to the surgery, which brought welcome relief.

The orthopedist failed to mention, however, that the operation would place considerable stress on the disks remaining. Normally, the lumbar spine has five disks that facilitate the movement of the lower back, with each one assuming approximately 20 percent of the flexing load. When a person bends, the disks—not the bones—must change shape and allow for flexibility. After Ruby's lowest lumbar disk was removed, she continued to bend as she always had except now *four* disks had to share the flexing function. Each had to carry a heavier burden, especially the one directly above the fused joint.

According to the *Encyclopedia of Medicine and Surgery*, after the two lower lumbar vertebrae have fused together, the disk above the fusion will most likely rupture in approximately seven years. Indeed, upon questioning Ruby, I discovered her problem recurred in about that length of time.

"I went back to my doctor," she said, "and he found another ruptured disk right above where he'd operated. He told me he should take it out just like the first one—after all, *that* surgery had been a success."

So the surgeon removed the disk between L4 and L5, and again Ruby recovered and felt relief. At that point, though, she had only *three* disks left to share the flexing load of the lower back, or 33 percent each. And as the encyclopedia article goes on to predict, the next higher disk ruptured five years later.

"Because the first two operations had worked," Ruby continued, "and I'd had twelve years without pain, the orthopedic surgeon suggested *another* one." Thus, he performed a third surgery on her lower back, removing the disk between L3 and L4, providing three additional pain-free years.

"But then when my neck started bothering me at the same time my back acted up again, I knew I had to try something else," she said.

It appeared the intricacies of spinal biomechanics had come into play: The long back muscles primarily support the spine in an upright position and maintain postural balance. Two such muscles—the *longissimus* and *spinalis*—start deep in the lower back, travel upward, and fasten to the vertebrae in the neck, without attaching to any other vertebrae on the way. Due to this phenomenon, known as "Lovett's half-wit brothers" in chiropractic circles,* abnormal stress in the lower back is reflected in the upper *cervical* (neck) region. As a result, the lowest lumbar vertebra, L5, is related to the top cervical vertebra, C1; L4 is related to C2; L3 to C3; L2 to C4; and L1 to C5.

Normally, the top of the third lumbar vertebra, L3, is parallel to the ground. Below L3, the fourth and fifth vertebrae, L4 and L5, pitch forward, and above L3, the first and second vertebrae, L1 and L2, pitch backward, producing the *lordosis* (swaybacked) curve. Ruby's lower three vertebrae had fused together, leaving L1 and L2 to assume all the bending stress. Because of their backward pitch, this load could no longer be transferred to the disks above L3 and had to be manifested elsewhere. According to Dr. Lovett, it would eventually show up in the neck.

"Alice raved about how you'd helped her, so I thought I'd come along and see if you could help me too."

"Well, I'll certainly do my best. Now, tell me about your pain—can you describe it?"

"Oh, I always hurt. Every time I move, I get twanging, shooting pains in my legs and butt as well as in my lower back. And sometimes I feel like my legs and feet are asleep."

---

*Named after Robert Lovett, M.D., a pioneer in medical research in the early 1900s.

"Have you had any numbness in your hands or arms like you've felt in your legs? That could happen with a neck problem because the nerves to the arms come from the neck."

"No, at least not yet. But considering how things have gone since I started with the surgeon, I wouldn't be surprised if it *did* happen."

"Are your activities limited in any way?"

"Yes, absolutely. I can hardly do anything without feeling bad. Just standing—like when I'm doing the dishes or the ironing—I get awfully tight and sore. The worst thing is vacuuming. It really kills my back, and then there's a pulling up into my neck. And I've had a tough time driving lately. When I look back over my shoulder, I get a terrible pain in my lower back. I don't drive much now—only when I absolutely have to. Alice is good about coming to pick me up if we're going somewhere."

At this point, I suggested taking x-rays to determine the exact state of Ruby's back. I took four views, all of them weight bearing. Generally, medical doctors take x-rays of the patient lying on a table top, whereas most chiropractic films are made with the patient standing upright to duplicate the posture of everyday activities.

The first two views were front and side (*A/P* and *lateral*), the standard practice for gaining the most information. I also needed to analyze the motion of the vertebral segments, so I took two more films from the front as Ruby bent over to each side as far as possible. Because her lower three vertebrae had presumably fused together, I wanted to determine how each vertebra functioned at the extremes of motion. (See chapter 12 to learn more about range of motion.)

To my surprise, I saw a small degree of separation between the vertebrae on the side opposite to the direction of bending—there *was* movement. The bones had not completely fused after all, which was a good sign. I finished by taking x-rays of Ruby's neck and studied the correlation between the half-wit brothers.

Next, I completed a thorough physical exam. As I suspected, her cervical and lumbar vertebrae had limited ranges of motion and were especially sore upon spinal palpation. I checked for and found weakness in the muscles that shared the same nerve supply as these vertebrae. Also, testing each area of the skin sharing that supply (a *dermatome*) revealed a reduction in sensation to temperature, touch, pain, or vibration.

Ruby showed every essential sign of neurological compromise in the lumbar area. Had she received chiropractic adjustments when her back pain first occurred, she may have been spared all of the surgeries and the resulting spinal deterioration.

After weighing my findings, including the fact that Ruby lived in Dodge City, Kansas, I told her, "This is what I suggest you do: Plan on three months of chiropractic care to see if I can return your spine to something close to normal. I propose setting daily appointments for the first week, and then you return to Dodge City for a week. I realize you can't stay in Boulder for several weeks at a time, but maybe after a few days at home, you can return for another week of intensive treatment?"

Ruby nodded. "I would sure like to try—as long as it's okay with my sisters. Alice would have to drive me, and we'd be staying here at June's place."

"See what you can arrange, and let me know if I can help. We'd go on an alternating schedule. One week of chiropractic adjustments and all other types of care—acupuncture, physical therapy, traction, nutritional supplements—and then a week at home doing self-care. After the fourth week of treatment, I'll reexamine you and we can decide if you've progressed enough to warrant continuing. You've got a lot of problems so I can't make any promises, but after a couple of months, we should be able to tell if chiropractic can help."

Ruby made plans to spend a week at her sister's in Arvada and then return as I'd recommended. Just as she was leaving that Friday for Kansas, I had an idea. "You know, Ruby, if you could possibly afford to buy a new vacuum cleaner, I'd strongly urge you to get an Oreck. We have one at home. It weighs only eight pounds and it's easy to push around. I think it'll spare your back."

Ten days later I saw Ruby again for another week of intensive treatment. "I've been having less pain," she said. "I'd really like to continue with your plan. Oh, and by the way, that Oreck really helped."

After six months of one-week-on and one-week-off care, Ruby was almost completely free of pain. Upon relocating to Utah, she sent me the following letter:

To Whom It May Concern:

I started going to Dr. Rude in June of 1974 when I lived in Dodge City, Kansas. My sister from Dodge City had seen Dr. Rude twice a day and stayed for a week of treatments for her arthritis. So I decided to give it a try. My back problems started back in the fifties. I had three lower vertebrae fused by an orthopedic surgeon. The trouble then moved to my neck. I also had extensive arthritis. Dr. Rude used spinal adjustments to correct the misalignments, rehabilitation and exercise to restore normal elasticity to the ligaments and to strengthen the muscles, acupuncture to balance my body's energy, ultrasound for the arthritis, pulsed diathermy to increase local circulation and metabolism, electrotherapy to stimulate the adrenal glands, and nutritional supplements to help normalize my body chemistry. Now my problems are all gone.

I have moved to Moab, Utah, but you can be certain that I will be telling people in Utah about Dr. Rude.

Ruby

P.S. Dr. Rude may use this letter as he sees fit.

28

Amanda's Herpes
Treating Skepticism, Headaches, and Cold Sores

> I see the body as more than just a collection of systems, organs, tissues, and fluids that independently break down or malfunction. I view the body as an integrated unit. No function of the body is independent of other functions.
>
> Ted Morter, D.C.
> Founder, B.E.S.T. Technique

One evening after her weekly bridge game, my wife, Shirley, burst into the house, seething. "There was a new woman at the club tonight named Helene," she said, barely inside the door. "Oscar Johnson married her last month—she's been married before and I guess she has a young daughter. Well! She had the gall to open her mouth and rake chiropractors over the coals, calling them quacks and accusing them of ripping off the public."

Shirley joined me in the living room and started marching back and forth, her fists clenched. I stood to greet her but then decided to retreat back to the safety of the couch.

"Of course, she *is* new to Hector—someone mentioned she's from Sacred Heart—and she didn't know I was a chiropractor's wife. She claims to be a registered nurse, so I suppose she considers herself an authority on health care. Huh! I heard her making terrible remarks like, 'I don't see how anyone can call them doctors.' It sure wasn't the time or place to set her straight, but I had a lot of trouble holding my tongue. It's a good thing we never sat at the same table—I know I couldn't have been civil to her." She suddenly stopped, let out a deep breath, and sank down next to me.

I put my arm around her and waited for her to calm down. "You know, Shirley, the ladies at the club who've been my patients will take her remarks with a grain of salt, and the others will just have to make up their own minds about what she said. I know that Doris and Barbara would have spoken up, but I'm sure they didn't want to embarrass her. I bet she'll feel very sheepish when she finds out you're married to me."

Considering Mrs. Johnson's outspoken display, imagine my surprise when I noticed her name in the appointment book a year later. I had not expected anyone who accepted the American Medical Association's anti-chiropractic propaganda to change her mind. Throughout the morning, I routinely adjusted patients, but all the while I kept wondering how I'd react when she and I were face to face.

Just before noon, after my receptionist, Jen, introduced her to me, Mrs. Johnson sat down across from me in my consultation room.

"I'm a registered nurse," she said, getting right to the point, "and I have never been to a chiropractor. In fact, because my education has been in the medical field, I know very little about chiropractic. But, I've had a severe headache for three and a half weeks, and Lorraine Schultz—she's a patient of yours who works with me at the hospital—says her headaches disappear when you crack her neck."

I listened to her trying to ease her mind about coming to see me, and at the same time, I assessed her posture, the way she carried her head relative to her shoulders and upper back, and the tilt of her head—one ear did appear to sit lower than the other. I also studied her head to see if I could detect any differences between the two sides of her face, indicating misaligned *cranial* (skull) bones that might be causing the pain. (See chapter 14 for information about cranial subluxations.)

"I've taken the usual over-the-counter remedies," she continued, "and when I was on duty at the hospital one night, I asked the doctor to give me a prescription for something stronger. It got rid of the headache, but when the drug wore off, the pain came back—it just won't let up. I've never believed in chiropractors, but Lorraine said, 'Go try him. You have nothing to lose.' So here I am. I get a lot of headaches, and this is the worst one I've ever had, so if you get rid of it, I'll be convinced chiropractic works."

At this point, I was chomping at the bit to lecture her on the effectiveness of spinal adjustments, but knowing that severe headaches are particularly painful and distracting, I decided to keep my mouth shut. Instead, I asked, "How long have you been suffering with these headaches?"

"I don't know—it's been years."

"How often do you have an attack like this?"

"At least once or twice a month, though they're usually not this severe. The last time I had a really bad one was maybe eight or nine months ago. I can manage pretty well with aspirin, but when it's like this, it's tough to do much of anything."

"Let's go find out the real cause of your problem." I led her to the examination room and handed her a gown. "Put this on with the opening in the back and lie face down on the table. I'll be back in a few minutes and we'll get started."

I've made it a habit to perform a "talking exam." I tell the patient exactly what I'm checking and the significance of my findings. I began palpating her neck and back musculature, and explained, "I'm finding a lot more muscle spasm on the right side than on the left." When I gently squeezed on her neck muscles, she told me she could feel the difference.

"This could cause headaches in a number of possible ways: Because muscles are designed to move bones, the uneven pull from these neck and back muscles could move the upper vertebrae enough to put pressure on the nerves, causing a headache." I moved slowly down her spine. "Or, the displaced vertebrae could be twisting the arteries that pass through them, partially obstructing blood flow and oxygen to the brain. And then another possibility is that the muscles fastened to the base of the skull are being tugged so hard that they're torquing the cranial bones, disrupting circulation in the head." I had decided that I just might be able to win her over by being very specific, drawing on her nursing training and familiarity with anatomy.

During the exam, I discovered the spinal segment T11 was extremely tender when I palpated it. "Were you aware of any soreness here?" I asked.

"No, not until you poked at it."

"This may be the source of the muscle tension that's distorting your spine. You see, as the spinal nerve emits from the spinal cord and passes laterally outward, it's actually three nerves wrapped up into one nerve sheath. One is a sensory nerve that carries messages from the skin to the brain, allowing you to feel temperature, moisture, pain, and the position of your body. The second nerve—the motor pathway—communicates with the muscles, which will contract only when they receive a message of stimulation. This T11 subluxation, or misalignment, could actually be stimulating the back muscles on the left side to contract out of proportion to the ones on the right. Let's go take some x-rays of your neck and back to find out what's going on."

"So what about the third nerve?" she asked as we walked back to the x-ray room. "What does it do?"

"That one belongs to the visceral branch and carries messages to the internal organs. The T11 nerve travels primarily to the kidneys."

"Do you mean to tell me that something out of place in my back could actually affect my kidneys? That is *really* hard to believe."

"Well, it certainly could."

"Hmm. . . . You know, now that I think about it, I *have* had to go to the bathroom a lot more often lately. I've even had to get up once in the middle of the night, which I can put up with—but not these headaches. So, my back could be causing *both* problems?"

"Yes, it's a good possibility."

After the x-rays confirmed subluxations in both the neck and lower *thoracic* (midback) areas, I outlined a treatment plan that included daily chiropractic adjustments until her headache disappeared. Then I adjusted T11 and the upper two *cervical* (neck) vertebrae.

"By gosh, I think you've helped me already." She smiled as she stood to leave. "The pain isn't nearly as strong as it was."

When Helene returned the next day, she looked more relaxed and less suspicious. "I read in my nursing textbooks about the things you talked about yesterday," she said. "I must admit your explanations were much easier to understand. And my headache is a lot better. I'm glad Lorraine Schultz sent me here."

"Please remember to thank Lorraine the next time you see her. And with respect to your headache, you know we haven't totally corrected the problem. You're feeling some relief, but your back isn't normal yet. After the headache clears completely, I'll reexamine you for subluxations by checking for muscle imbalance or pain. We won't stop until we return everything to normal—chiropractors go beyond just removing the pain or symptoms."

On her third visit, Helene told me her headache was practically gone. "It does come back just a bit," she said, "but then it goes away again. I suppose my movements throughout the day shift the vertebrae slightly and the headache returns. And when they slip back into place, the pain goes away."

"It's more complex than that, but you've got the gist of it," I said, palpating her spine. "The various muscles supporting the neck originate from a number of areas in the shoulders, ribs, and lower vertebrae. The *longissimus dorsi*, for example, begins on the five lower vertebrae just above the pelvis and runs up the back where it fastens at the top five cervical vertebrae in the neck, without attaching to any other vertebrae along the way (see chapter 27 for further details). It's possible for a subluxation in your lower back to exert forces on the neck, so if you happen to move just right—or *wrong*—you'll develop a crick in your neck."

I asked her to turn over on her back. "I've been thinking a lot about chiropractic," she said, "and how it seems to comply with nature." She paused while I adjusted her neck. "I've been wondering—is chiropractic effective for treating conditions other than headaches, and neck and back problems? And how safe is it?"

"To answer your first question—chiropractic has had miraculous results in a number of non-back-related cases. And as far as safety goes, one of the chiropractic colleges checked all the records of patients who had received adjustments by student interns over the school's history, and they didn't find one fatality associated with chiropractic treatment. I don't know how many years that covered, but they looked at over one million adjustments."

"Well, that's really good to hear." We were finished for the day and she stood up to leave. "Oh, two more things—can children get out of alignment? And can they be adjusted?"

"Yes, to both questions. How about bringing in your kids for a complimentary exam?"

That's how I met nine-year-old Amanda, or Mandy, as everyone called her, and her baby brother, Curtis. When they first arrived with their mother, I took Mandy's hand and led her to the collection of coloring books and toys I kept in my reception room. I wanted to give her some time to feel comfortable before examining her spine.

Jen helped me with Curtis, who was a tiny bundle of smiles. He seemed to think we were playing a game, making it easy to examine him.

"This little guy's spine checks out fine, Helene, though neck subluxations can easily develop during delivery. When the mother bears down to push, she exerts a tremendous compression force on the baby. Or, consider a forceps delivery, when the doctor pulls on a tiny infant's neck to extract it. A baby's neck was not designed to be in traction."

When it was Mandy's turn, she hung back, apprehensive. Doctor visits for her meant getting shots, and I'm sure she didn't relish being examined by a new doctor. Fortunately, I had delved into magic as a teenager. "Here, Mandy, look," I said. "I have nothing in my right hand and nothing in my left. But, hey, what's this?" I deftly pulled a nickel out of her ear and gave it to her. "This must belong to you because I don't have any nickels in my hands or pockets."

Her face lit up. She turned and handed the coin to her mom. "Could you please keep this for me, so I can put it in my bank when we get home?"

Relaxed now, Mandy jumped up on the table and I checked her spine. I discovered a moderate degree of spasm in the muscles on the left side of her neck as well as in those running along the right side of her thoracic spine.

I placed Helene's hand on her daughter's neck and told her to lightly palpate the area. "This spasm will not cause any pain or obvious difficulty," I said. "It isn't severe enough to change her posture or make her carry her head bent to one side, although it will eventually distort her spine. I can't predict the future, but I do check my son Carlton's back at least twice a month."

Helene gave me the go-ahead to adjust her daughter. "Every time I come in here I learn something new about chiropractic," she said. "I'm really impressed with how effective it is for so many things."

There's an old saying, "A man convinced against his will is of the same opinion still." The reverse is also true—when a person holding a strong belief is convinced by the facts to do an about face, the new view is held just as strongly. So it was with Helene. She continued under chiropractic care and regularly had her children examined. She brought in her husband, "Buzz" (Oscar's nickname), and a couple of years later, another son, Andy. She referred many to my office; in fact, patients drove forty miles from Sacred Heart to Hector because Helene was continuously spreading the word about chiropractic.

The members of the Johnson family seldom missed their regular monthly appointments, giving me the chance to watch the children grow and mature. When Mandy turned twelve and the typical adolescent hormones began to rage, I had a discussion with her and her mother about the chemical changes taking place. I gave them a list of dietary dos and don'ts for avoiding complexion problems and recommended nutritional supplements for smoothing out the emotional highs and lows.

And then shortly after graduating from Hector High, Mandy married Ross Donaldson, who became a patient too. I remember one blustery winter day, about a year after her wedding, when Mandy came to my office. "I've got *another* cold sore," she complained. "They're really painful—I'm tired of getting them all the time."

On the right side of her face, I saw a large fever blister, starting from the crease where the lips come together, traveling up over her upper lip, and reaching almost to the lower edge of the right nostril. Seeping out of it was a light, yellowish liquid. The sore looked raw and painful.

I told Mandy the infections are caused by the virus *herpes simplex*.

"Well, I kiss Ross and he doesn't get them. Why do I?"

"Some people tend to be more prone than others to developing blisters," I said. "Let me try to explain with a brief chemistry lesson: *Calcium bicarbonate* is a substance in the body that helps maintain the acid-base balance, which is important for good health. If the level of calcium bicarbonate is inadequate—as I suspect is happening with you—this delicate balance is disturbed, making the skin tissues vulnerable to the sores produced by the herpes virus."

She seemed to be following me so I continued, "Now, for the tougher part: Each calcium bicarbonate molecule is the combination of a negative bicarbonate *radical*, or subunit, and a positive calcium radical. The bicarbonate part is formed when carbon dioxide reacts with water. Considering our bodies contain 65 percent water and constantly produce carbon dioxide, we have a steady supply of raw materials to create ample bicarbonate. That means, then, that there's probably a lack of calcium in the tissue fluids to combine with the bicarbonate."

"So how do I get more calcium where it needs to be?"

"With these supplements," I said, handing Mandy three bottles. "The *calcium lactate* provides calcium; the *betaine hydrochloride* supplies additional stomach acidity, which helps break down the calcium so it'll cross the stomach membranes into the blood more easily; and *Cataplex F*, a Standard Process supplement, diffuses calcium from the blood stream into the skin tissues."

Cataplex F contains the essential fatty acid *alpha linolenic*, a derivative of flaxseed oil. In addition to diffusing calcium into the tissues, essential fatty acids (EFAs) help maintain the integrity of the skin, hair, nails, nerves, and brain tissue. And because of their important relationship to iodine metabolism, they may participate in regulating thyroid function. EFAs also support the immune system and enhance the effects of vitamin D and B-6, the latter being essential to normal female hormone production. Furthermore, research has shown they are beneficial in the treatment of prostate disorders.

(The "F" is a throwback to when scientists first discovered vitamins and started identifying them with the letters of the alphabet. Besides the now-familiar vitamins A, B, C, D, and E, several other vitamins—F, G, H, and so forth—were also identified. Eventually, someone realized that vitamin G and those following it had much in common with vitamin B and lumped them altogether as B Complex: vitamin B became known as B-1, G as B-2, H as B-3, and so forth. Although the old nomenclature "vitamin F" is generally no longer used, Standard Process chose to retain it.)

At Mandy's appointment the next day, I noticed the herpes lesion had dried up, leaving a crusty scab behind. She told me it wasn't nearly as tender. And three days later when I checked her again, the cold sore wasn't even visible. "That's the best, fastest relief I've ever had," she said.

"I assume the Cataplex F was the most important supplement of the three I gave you. Considering you drink plenty of milk—which is a good source of calcium lactate—and at age twenty you're producing adequate stomach acid, it looks like your body needed help spreading calcium into the skin tissues."

"Well, why don't I just take it on a regular basis? If you're right about what it does with the calcium, I won't have any more cold sores."

I nodded. "Sounds like a good idea."

Mandy came to see me for her regular appointments several more times before I moved to Colorado. She occasionally picked up a bottle of Cataplex F but never mentioned cold sores again.

Author's Note:

I cared for Helene and her family for many years. They had no health challenges, the children had perfect school attendance, and they did not consult with any other doctor.

One day Helene really surprised me. "You know, Buzz makes enough from farming that I don't have to work—I just like taking care of sick people. If Mrs. Anderson ever quits working for you, would you consider hiring me as your assistant?"

I'm sure she would have been a valuable asset to the Rude Chiropractic Center in Hector; however, Mrs. Anderson was with me until I left for Colorado.

29

Samantha's Sciatica
Delving Deeper to Find the Cause

> Our nature consists in motion; complete rest is death.
> *Blaise Pascal*
> *(1623–1662)*

Every year the Boulder College of Massage awards diplomas to students longing to earn a living using the skills they've mastered. Some graduates return to their roots in other states, while many choose to stay in Boulder, possibly because of the desirable climate or the unique cultural and educational environment. Those who remain usually mail out letters of introduction to all health-care practitioners announcing they're open for business. Samantha Martin went one step further and actually made appointments to meet with the doctors, at which time she offered a complimentary massage.

Despite her petite size—just four feet nine and under a hundred pounds—Samantha had the strength required to effectively work a client's musculature. After giving me an excellent massage, I referred a number of my patients to her, and her business grew steadily.

Single when we first met, Samantha sent out wedding announcements about six months later. And then the following year, her name appeared in my appointment book.

"You remember that I got married?" she said when I asked her how she was doing. "Well, now I'm pregnant, and I've been having this terrible pain for a while—it runs down the back of my left leg. I thought chiropractic might help me."

"How far along is your pregnancy?" I noticed she was starting to show.

"Almost five months."

"Hmm. All the nerves emitting from the lumbar area and through the openings in the sacrum—the *sciatic nerves*—travel down the back of the leg. You must have something going on in your lower back that's putting pressure on those nerves and causing pain."

I told her I wouldn't be taking x-rays because the radiation could be harmful to the baby. (I think back to when Shirley was pregnant with our two boys, and it was a common medical practice at that time.) "So it'll be a little more difficult to pinpoint the exact cause of your problem."

I decided to depend on my skill in palpating the spine and some *kinesiological testing* to find the exact area needing attention. In his 1972 workshop manual, *Applied Kinesiology*, George Goodheart, D.C., explains that certain muscles receive their dominant nerve supply from specific neurological levels of the spine. By testing the strength of these muscles and comparing the right and left sides, I could possibly identify a weak muscle—and the corresponding level of the spine causing some interference—and hone in on the problem.

I directed Samantha to lie face up on the adjusting table. I began by checking the *extensor hallucis longus*, the muscle responsible for bending the big toe toward the head. Her left toe was weaker than the right one, but without the usual weakness I would have expected. The fifth lumbar nerve supplies this muscle as well as the uterus and is part of the sciatic nerve that runs down the back of the leg.

Next, I tested the muscle involved in bending the foot toward the head, the *tibialis anterior*. This is supplied by the fourth lumbar nerve, another branch of the sciatic nerve, which also supplies the colon. Both sides tested strong. The remaining branches of the sciatic nerve come from the sacral nerves, and their conditions cannot be determined through muscle testing.

Even though her big toe's strength was not severely diminished, I had nothing else to "hang my hat on," so that's where I started.

"You know, Samantha, I'm not a hundred percent sure I've found the problem, but I'll give you an adjustment and see how you feel." I instructed her to turn over face down, and when I palpated her fifth lumbar vertebra—the area through which the fifth lumbar nerve emits—she complained about some discomfort, indicating a possible subluxation.

For additional verification, I palpated the *atlas* (the top vertebra in the neck), or C1, and discovered minor tenderness on the right side. By using the Sacro-Occipital Technique (SOT),* D.C.'s can determine the presence and location of a misalignment based on the relationship between the *cervical* (neck) and lumbar vertebrae. C1, the highest vertebra, can provide information about L5, the lowest vertebra. The C1 tenderness indicated that L5 was rotated back on the opposite side. This situation actually begins with a change in L5's position, causing an unequal tension between the left and right muscles that begins in the lumbar area and travels up to the neck.

After directing Samantha to lie on her right side and bend her left leg, I adjusted her fifth lumbar with a backward thrust.

"Oh, it didn't work—the pain is still there," she said.

At this point, I decided to use my knowledge of acupuncture to temporarily ease her symptoms. Two major acupuncture points on the body can be needled to bring relief to a patient suffering from sciatica pain: *Huan Tiao*, or *Gall Bladder 30* (GB30), located behind the *greater trochanter* (the large rounded part of the thigh bone protruding out at the upper part of the hip) and in the middle of the deep hollow that is formed while standing erect with muscles tensed; and *Wei Zhong*, or *Bladder 54* (UB54), found in the center of the fold in the back of the knee. When I inserted the needles, Samantha experienced some relief almost instantly, and as time elapsed, the discomfort lessened even more.

"Acupuncture will help with the pain," I said, "but if we don't correct the cause, it'll come back again."

Samantha left the office feeling much better, although the very next day she called to tell me her pain had returned. "Maybe not as bad as it was yesterday but almost," she said. "I'll see you this afternoon."

We were able to control the pain with daily chiropractic and acupuncture treatments, yet we weren't making any progress. Then, over

---

*Founded by Dr. Major B. DeJarnette, this technique is one of the various chiropractic methods available for determining the presence and location of a spinal misalignment. It is based upon examining the tension of the postural muscles the body uses to maintain an upright position.

two weeks later, she asked me, "Did I tell you that I slipped on the ice a couple of months ago? Could that have caused my problem?"

"When you slipped, did you come down hard on your butt?"

"Yes, I sure did. My feet went right out from under me, and I landed hard on my left cheek."

"That may be the key," I said. "You see, the baby begins to grow from the moment of fertilization. At twelve to thirteen weeks, it should be about two and a half to three inches long—maybe about the size of a swollen thumb. Normally, the uterus lies in a position that's almost parallel to the ground. When you fell and hit your backside, the uterus could have shifted perpendicular to its usual position. It's possible the fetus had enough bulk to flop backward causing the uterus to flip backward also—what we call a *retroverted uterus*. The baby is then developing behind where it's supposed to be, and as it grows, it presses on the sacral branches of the sciatic nerves. How long after the fall did your leg pain start?"

"Well, I don't remember exactly—maybe a month ago. It kept getting worse until you did the acupuncture."

"It's reasonable to believe that your fall caused a retroversion of the uterus and now it's pressing on the sacral nerves on the left side. I suggest we do a pelvic exam to find out." Chiropractors are taught to examine the female reproductive system in the same manner as medical doctors.

Without hesitating, she said, "Okay, let's do it."

During the exam, the doctor inserts his finger into the vagina and palpates the neck of the uterus. The rounded part of the uterus (*fundus*) should rest up toward the pubic bone. Instead, I felt it leaning backward and resting back against the front side of the sacrum. I brought out my anatomy books to show her what was normal and then drew a picture to illustrate her situation. I also demonstrated it on a pelvis specimen I use to explain anatomy to my patients.

"Samantha, I have to tell you that this will make the delivery very difficult if it's not corrected. Your medical doctor would most likely have to perform a cesarean."

"Can it *be* corrected?" she asked, sounding worried.

"I can manipulate the uterus from the inside, but the more effective treatment is an exercise I'll teach you." I manually tried flipping the fundus back to its normal position. "Now, for the exercise: Get down on all fours, not on your knees, but on your hands and feet, with your rear end way up in the air. Walk around the house in that position for at least five minutes. You must do it three or four times every day." By moving on all fours with her pelvis in this unusual position, her uterus could fall forward into its normal location. "Try it now so I can make sure you know how to do it."

Samantha moved down to the floor and started laughing as she did the exercise around the room. Just before she left the office, she turned to me and said, "I think it feels better already."

Throughout the rest of her pregnancy, Samantha continued doing the exercise and receiving chiropractic care, and eventually her sciatic pains disappeared. She delivered a beautiful baby girl—after only about *three hours* of labor.

Samantha brought her daughter, Michelle, into the office when she was just a month old. I didn't see her again until her mother returned for an appointment more than three years later. "I had such an easy time when Michelle was born," Samantha told me, "and now that I'm pregnant again, I want to have regular adjustments from the very beginning."

I remember at one of her visits, Samantha brought Michelle along and pointed out a photo I had on the wall showing me in the water with a dolphin. I had recently taken a cruise from Los Angeles down the west coast of Mexico. When we stopped at Puerto Vallarta, I took a side trip to an aquarium and swam with the dolphins, and the director shot the picture of me. "Look, there's Dr. Rude kissing a dolphin," Samantha said. Little Michelle stood there, her mouth wide open and eyes as big as saucers, and then looked up at me and asked, "Did it kiss you back?"

30

Water in the Ear, Broken Ribs, and Sunburn
Seeing Is Believing

> Chiropractors are the most qualified physicians. Their training includes everything a medical doctor learns, except how to prescribe drugs and perform surgery, but they learn body chemistry and nutrition, all means of natural healing and physical therapies, and some specialize in radiology, orthopedics, sports injuries, and spinal rehabilitation.
>
> *Wally Unruh, D.C.*

A couple of years after my wife, Shirley, passed away, I met Jeannie at the Boulder Social Singles Club. We discovered we had a lot in common, particularly our devotion to our families. Her four children and my two sons live in California, and in 1999 we started traveling together to see them. Jeannie and I grew close, and the following year we exchanged wedding vows. Without a doubt, I am truly blessed to have met and married two wonderful women.

In September 1999 Jeannie and I visited her son Kent in South Pasadena. Soon after we arrived, he told us his right ear had been bothering him. "I guess I'm going to have to go see the doctor," he said. "I've had this weird feeling in my ear for almost two weeks. I keep thinking it'll go away, but it's still there, so I better get it checked out."

His complaint made me remember a lecture given by Dr. Major B. DeJarnette, the originator of the Sacro-Occipital Technique (see chapter 29). He maintained that a slipped *sacroiliac joint*—the area joining the *sacrum* (the seat bone at the base of the spine) and the *ilium* (hip bone)—can cause a sensation of water in the ear. I'd never actually had a patient with this problem, but that didn't stop me. "Does it feel like you've got water in your ear?" I asked.

"Well, sort of . . . yes, now that you mention it, that's a good way to describe it, though I haven't been to the beach in months."

I hesitated before proceeding. I knew that Jeannie had gone to a chiropractor only once in her teens; otherwise, like many others, she had raised her family under the care of a traditional medical doctor. Over the previous year or so, I had been gradually teaching her about chiropractic and adjustments, but I hadn't as yet treated her children.

"You know, Kent, you may have a slipped sacroiliac joint, which can sometimes cause that kind of sensation in the ear. Do you have a place where you can lie flat on your back but up off the floor? If you don't mind, I'd like to check some things."

"I have a weight bench in the rec room. Will that work?"

"Perfect."

The three of us went downstairs, and I told Kent to lie down on the bench with his legs straight out. In this position—lying face up on a hard surface—the length of the legs will not appear to be the same length if the sacroiliac joint has moved out of alignment. When I compared Kent's legs, I discovered his right leg was almost a half inch shorter than his left. (This examination cannot be performed on a bed because the body's weight will sink into the mattress and negate the results.)

I moved to the head of the bench and faced him. "Now, I'd like to check your arm strength. Stay lying down and raise both hands to the ceiling. I'm going to try to push your hands toward your feet. Keep your elbows stiff and push back against me. Don't let me move your arms."

Kent's right arm gave way—another positive sign for a sacroiliac subluxation. This arm-strength test was developed by Dr. George Goodheart, who expanded this form of muscle testing into a technique known as *applied kinesiology*, a diagnostic tool often used by chiropractors.

Then I palpated the *anterior superior iliac spine* of both hip bones (the bony prominence on the front of each hip bone just below the waist, frequently referred to as a "hip-pointer" in athletic circles), and Kent told me the right one was definitely tender—the third indicator of a sacroiliac problem. Finally, I checked the *sartorius muscle*, located on the inside of the leg just below the knee, which helps stabilize the sacroiliac joint. Again, the right side was tender. The results of all four tests confirmed my initial diagnosis.

"Kent, just as I thought, your sacroiliac is misaligned. If you let me adjust your spine, I think I can remove that water-in-the-ear feeling."

He looked up at his mother, who nodded, and then he turned back to me. "Go ahead," he said, sounding uncertain. I sensed he may have agreed only to avoid upsetting Jeannie.

"While you're lying there, I'm going to feel the back of your neck. When there's a sacroiliac problem, there's usually a *cervical*, or neck, vertebra out of alignment as well."

I palpated his neck and found some soreness on the right *transverse process of the atlas* (the bony structure of the top cervical vertebra). After placing my hands on this area, I carefully turned his head to the left and thrust. A loud popping filled the air.

"Whoa! What was that?" Kent's hands flew to his neck.

"That's normal," I said, regretting not having prepared him better. "The vertebrae make that kind of sound when they move back into their proper positions."

I rubbed his neck and let him relax before continuing. "Okay, now we're going to fix your sacroiliac, and you'll probably hear the same sound. Lie on your left side," I directed, moving to the side of the bench. "Bend your right leg and lift it to about my waist level." With my left hand, I contacted the *posterior superior iliac spine* of the right hip bone (the hard part of the hip bone that protrudes out of the back) and then pressed his right shoulder back with my other hand to torque his spine. Again, we heard a popping as I adjusted the errant joint, but this time Kent remained calm.

"We're done. Roll onto your back, and let me check things again." His legs were now the same length. "Good. Now, raise your arms to the ceiling." I tried pushing them toward his feet as I had before, but both arms stayed strong and upright.

Kent's face brightened as he realized I had somehow changed his body. "Geez, those two cracking noises really made a difference."

I helped him sit up on the edge of the weight bench and told him to stand up. As he rose, he shrugged his shoulders and arched his back, testing his mobility. He twisted left and right at his hips, and then rolled his head first one way and then the other.

"That feels great," he said. "I'm all loosened up."

"And how is that feeling in your ear now?"

"My ear? Uh . . . it's gone. It's *all gone*." His eyes widened in surprise. "Amazing. I went around with that miserable feeling in my ear for two weeks, and within just a few minutes you got rid of it—just like that." He snapped his fingers. "Absolutely amazing. I can't get over how simple and fast it was." He smiled and shook my hand.

Shortly thereafter, I took off for the other side of Pasadena and spent the night with my son and his children.

The next morning, Jeannie called, panicked. "I'm so glad you're there! Kent fell at work and may have broken some ribs. He's on his way home. Can you come over right away?"

I hurried to the other side of town and pulled up behind Kent just as he turned into the driveway. Jeannie must have been watching for him because she raced outside, and the two of us helped him into the house.

"I was taking down this huge antique mirror," he said, struggling to talk. "Very ornate, with a heavy metal frame. Must weigh close to two hundred pounds." He paused to take a breath, wincing. "I had it in my arms, and as I was backing down the ladder, I slipped—landed on a display case. It looks like nothing broke—except maybe me. I felt something crack inside my ribs."

"Let me help you take off your shirt," I said. "I want to listen to your chest." Having no stethoscope, I pressed my ear to the area on his back where he said the pain was the worst. (After all, doctors used their ears long before stethoscopes were invented.) "Take a deep breath and let it out slowly. Tell me if the pain gets worse or better at any time." If he had fractured ribs, I might have been able to hear an abnormal clicking or grating noise as the broken ends rubbed over each other.

Just then the telephone interrupted us. An employee was calling from Anthropologie, the upscale store Kent manages, to tell him to go to the emergency room. According to workers' compensation rules, an accident report had been filled out and faxed to company headquarters. Word came back that Kent needed to get x-rays immediately.

I continued with the exam but found nothing. "I don't hear anything that would confirm there's a break, Kent. The cracking could have been similar to the sound you heard when I adjusted your back. The rib heads may have been changing positions in the joints at the spine. I suggest we go and have an x-ray taken anyway. Considering it's a workers' comp case, you should get an x-ray for your own protection—just in case it *is* something serious."

Kent nodded his agreement and Jeannie grabbed his shirt to help him put it on.

"Before you get dressed," I said, "it might help to bind up your midsection. If a rib *is* broken, as you breathe and your chest expands and contracts, the end of the bone could change position and irritate the site of the fracture. Do you have any dish towels?" Back when I was teaching first aid for the American Red Cross, I showed students how to bind fractured ribs with the standard cloth square from a first aid kit. Kent didn't own ordinary thin dish towels, so Jeannie and I had to improvise with one of his old shirts.

We piled into the car, and I drove us to the Huntington Medical Center. "They'll probably take several x-rays in different positions," I explained on the way, "because it's difficult to see a broken rib. To view any fracture easily, the broken ends must be displaced from each other enough for the x-rays to pass between them. But ribs don't usually break that way—they're more like green-stick fractures. If the doctor doesn't find any positive proof either way, he may tell you to come back in a week and get another x-ray. During that time, if there has been a break, the damaged cells on the open ends of each bone fragment will be absorbed, and new ones that are rich in calcium will take their place. The follow-up x-ray will clearly show the new calcium."

At the hospital, Kent completed the paperwork, and a nurse escorted him in to see a doctor. Almost two hours later, Kent reappeared and explained, "You were right. They did take quite a few x-rays and from various angles. I sat there and waited while they were being processed, and just as you predicted, the doctor told me they were inconclusive. I'm supposed to go back in a week."

Back at Kent's house, Jeannie and I again helped him inside.

"Kenn, should I put hot or cold on my ribs?" He slowly sank down onto the couch.

"Don't put hot on it for the first day. Heat will draw blood into the area, and if there's been any damage to blood vessels from the accident, it could cause more bleeding. Cold will constrict the tiny capillaries and reduce the swelling—so use cold."

The next day, Jeannie and I headed back to Colorado.

A week later, Kent called to let us know he had indeed cracked his ribs, but they were healing and the pain was slowly going away. Then one morning about a month after that, I received a surprise phone call at the office.

"Mom told me to give you a call," Kent said. "She said you'd probably be able to help. The big boss had decided we should hold a staff meeting on the beach in Malibu, combining business with pleasure, and maybe even do a little surfing."

"Sounds like a lot of fun."

"Well, it *was*, but now I've got one whale of a sunburn—all over my back and shoulders. Do you have any magic remedy for someone who looks like a lobster?"

"Yes, as a matter of fact, I do," I answered, pleased he called for my advice. "Go to any health food store and ask for a bottle of unsaturated essential fatty acids. Take six times the dosage recommended on the bottle. It's a high dose, but your body can tolerate it on a one-time basis. Call tomorrow and let us know what happened."

The next afternoon, Jeannie called me at the office. "Kent said the soreness left in about a half hour, and this morning he was as brown as a nice piece of mahogany furniture."

Up until just a few short weeks before, Kent had experienced only traditional medical care. After seeing that I was able to solve his ear complaint and advise him on the proper care of fractured ribs, he started believing and trusting in chiropractic—so much so that he called looking for a solution to a condition that most people would have let time heal. Alternative health care offers a multitude of simple, safe answers. All you have to do is ask.

Epilogue

I have enjoyed sharing these narratives with you and hope you have gained as much from reading them as I have from recalling and recounting them.

In closing, I present a short poem written by R. Lee Sharpe many decades ago. These words have always served as a sort of beacon, guiding me whenever I needed a moment to reflect upon some troubling situation:

> *Isn't it strange how princes and kings,*
> *And clowns that caper in sawdust rings,*
> *And common people, like you and me,*
> *Are builders of eternity?*
>
> *Each is given a list of rules;*
> *A shapeless mass, a bag of tools.*
> *And each must fashion, ere life is flown,*
> *A stumbling block, or a stepping stone.*

I encourage you to look upon *Healing Miracles Great and Small* as a stepping stone, one that leads to better health and a longer, more fulfilling life for you, your family, and your friends.

GOD BLESS YOU.

Appendix
Laboratories and Supplement Distributors

The specific products and laboratories mentioned within this book are not connected with its production. The addresses, telephone numbers, and Web sites listed below are subject to change. Please note that all products are sold only through health-care professionals.

Anabolic Laboratories
Nutritional and herbal formulations
Lake Forest, CA
800-445-6849
www.anaboliclabs.com

Apex Energetics
Homeopathic and nutritional formulas
16592 Hale Ave.
Irvine, CA 92606
800-736-4381
www.apexenergetics.com

Dartell Laboratories
3300 Hyland Avenue
Costa Mesa, CA 714-545-0100

Foot Levelers, Inc.
Flexible, custom-made orthotics
P.O. Box 12611
Roanoke, VA 24027-2611
www.footlevelers.com

NutriWest
Nutritional supplements
P.O. Box 950
Douglas, WY 82633
800-443-3333
www.nutriwest.com

Standard Process
Whole food supplements
Palmyra, Wisconsin
1-800-558-8740
www.standardprocess.com

Systemic Formulas, Inc.
Wonder Oil
High-quality supplements
P.O. Box 1516
Ogden, UT 84402
1-800-445-4647
www.systemicformulas.com

Complimentary Chiropractic Visit

Anyone who has obtained a new copy of *Healing Miracles Great and Small* is entitled to one complimentary chiropractic consultation and examination (x-rays may not be included). Simply call a D.C. in your area, and mention this book and offer when making an appointment. In the event a doctor does not wish to participate, choose another practitioner.

At the beginning of your visit, present this page to the chiropractor, and at the end, he or she can complete and sign the short form below.

If you or your doctor has health questions (not all chiropractors are familiar with every protocol I have described), or you would like to share ideas or comments about this book, please contact me at drkennonrudedc@aol.com. Also, if you have difficulty finding a chiropractor in your area, send me an e-mail and I will do my best to locate one for you.

I wrote *Healing Miracles Great and Small* to educate readers on the benefits of alternative health care. Estimates indicate that more than 50 percent of the American people have never seen a Doctor of Chiropractic. I urge you to use this free offer to improve that figure—and more importantly, your health.

I, _____, have provided one complimentary
          Chiropractor's Name

chiropractic consultation to _____.
                                                  Patient's Name

Today's Date: _____

Chiropractor's Signature: _____

ISBN 1412034671